BALANCE EXERCISES
FOR SENIORS

ILLUSTRATED & EASY TO FOLLOW GUIDE WITH BEGINNER 5-10 MINUTE HOME EXERCISES FOR SENIORS FOR EXCELLENT STABILITY, POSTURE & FALL PREVENTION.

PROVEN 30 DAY WORKOUT PLAN

JOHN WILLIAMSON

TABLE OF CONTENTS

• EXPLANATION OF CAUSES & SYMPTOMS OF LOSS OF BALANCE & WHAT TO DO ABOUT IT TO BECOME STURDY AS A ROCK ... **P 3**

• THE LATEST SCIENTIFIC RESEARCH ON IMPROVING STABILITY & BALANCE .... **P 6**

• HOW TO ASSESS YOUR CURRENT STABILITY AND BALANCE LEVELS .... **P 9**

• IDENTIFYING AREAS OF WEAKNESS AND IMBALANCE & HOW TO QUICKLY IMPROVE THEM .... **P 11**

• DANGERS OF LACK OF STABILITY & HOW TO PREVENT THEM FOR GOOD .... **P 13**

• 4 BIGGEST MISTAKES SENIORS MAKE THAT PREVENT THEM FROM BEING MORE STABLE ON THEIR FEET .... **P 15**

• FOOD & SUPPLEMENTS RECOMMENDED BY EXPERTS FOR IMPROVED BALANCE & STABILITY .... **P 19**

• STEP BY STEP STATIC BALANCE EXERCISES FOR IMPROVED POSTURE & BALANCE .... **P 21**

• STEP BY STEP DYNAMIC BALANCE EXERCISES FOR IMPROVED BALANCE & COORDINATION .... **P 31**

• STEP BY STEP PROPRIOCEPTIVE EXERCISES TO ENHANCE SENSORY AWARENESS & BALANCE CONTROL .... **P 42**

• STEP BY STEP BALANCE-FOCUSED CARDIO EXERCISES FOR IMPROVED CARDIOVASCULAR HEALTH & STABILITY .... **P 50**

• FALL PREVENTION STRATEGIES FOR REDUCING FALL RISK IN DAILY LIFE & LIVING SAFELY .... **P 57**

• STEP BY STEP ADVANCED EXERCISES TO IMPROVE STABILITY AND BALANCE .... **P 63**

• PROGRESSION AND MAINTENANCE STRATEGIES TO KEEP GOING & STICK TO YOUR NEW HABITS .... **P 71**

Explanation of causes & symptoms of loss of balance & what to do about it to become sturdy as a rock

Balance is a fundamental aspect of functioning from day to day, and it's one of those things that you never really think about – until you start to struggle. Most of us learn to balance as infants, and rarely need to consider the skill again, except occasionally. We do utilise our balance every day, when doing things like riding bikes, walking around, and even just standing upright, but we don't often think about it.

However, many of us also find that our balance worsens as we age, and we start to struggle with things like bending, leaning, and lifting. You might notice this in little moments, like if you stand on one foot to clean your other foot in the shower, or while you're putting your socks on at the start of the day. You may never have had very good balance, even as a child, or you might just find that your balance is deteriorating as you age.

Regardless, not being able to balance well can be a scary feeling. What seems easy most of the time suddenly becomes challenging, and you find yourself at risk of stumbling onto the floor and hurting yourself. It's never fun to feel like you aren't steady on your feet, and this comes with a serious risk of falls. It can rob you of your independence, resulting in increased dependence on loved ones or other support services.

Lack of balance can also reduce your confidence, making you feel unsafe, and making it harder for you to do things – which can reduce your balance even further if you are discouraged from being physically active. It may have a major impact on your quality of life, and the things you are able to do each day.

Some of the symptoms of lack of balance include:

- Staggering when you're trying to walk
- Confusion
- Feeling like you are going to fall over
- Blurry vision
- A spinning sensation (vertigo/dizziness)
- Disorientation
- Falling over
- Feeling faint

A lot of people dismiss mild balance problems as just part of life and a normal part of ageing, but doing so can be dangerous. You need to make sure you address balance problems before they result in a fall, especially if you have other health conditions, such as osteoporosis.

Part of that often involves looking at what's causing the lack of balance. Some people naturally have poor balance (although there are still things you can do to improve it), but other things can cause this, such as:

- CERTAIN MEDICATIONS
- EYE MUSCLE IMBALANCE
- HEAD INJURIES
- MIGRAINES
- MENIERE'S DISEASE
- INNER EAR PROBLEMS
- NEUROLOGICAL CONDITIONS
- INJURIES

- LOW BLOOD PRESSURE OR HIGH BLOOD PRESSURE
- EAR INFECTIONS
- MUSCLE WEAKNESS
- MOTION SICKNESS
- POOR BLOOD CIRCULATION
- AGEING
- CHEMICAL IMBALANCES IN THE BRAIN

There are plenty of other things that can also cause balance problems, but those are some of the commonest. It's important to address any sudden changes in your balance with your doctor, because poor balance is often linked with medical issues. Get checked out for health problems before you do anything else. Don't just work on improving your balance without finding out if there's a reason it isn't good.

Your doctor may offer advice specific to your situation that will help to address the issue. For example, if you have an inner ear infection, they will provide treatment. If you have eye problems or blood pressure problems, they may be able to provide medications that will help.

However, even if you have an underlying condition and it gets treated, you can still benefit from reading this book. Everybody can improve their balance and enjoy increased confidence and reduced fall risks as a result!

Exercise is one of the best and most effective ways to tackle poor balance. By strengthening your core muscles, you give yourself a much better chance of staying upright and firmly on your feet – so that's what we're going to look at throughout this book.

Although balance exercises are often associated with older individuals, anybody can benefit from improving their balance, and you can certainly get value from this book even if you're young. With that in mind, let's start looking at the balance exercises you might want to try.

THE LATEST SCIENTIFIC RESEARCH ON IMPROVING STABILITY & BALANCE

WHAT DOES SCIENCE TELL US ABOUT IMPROVING OUR BALANCE?

It is thought that our sense of balance starts to deteriorate very early in life. Estimates vary, but some studies have suggested it could be as early as the age of 25. At this point, you've reached the peak of your physical performance, and your physical activity may start to drop off, among other changes. Many individuals don't notice for a long time that they are becoming less good at balancing. It is often not until an individual is 60 or older that they start to realise they are not as stable on their feet as they used to be. That's good news in some ways – you may not have to deal with this problem much when you are young – but it also means that you may neglect your balancing muscles and fail to work on your balance until you're a senior.

A lot of studies in recent years have pointed to the importance of exercise when it comes to improving your balance. Many of these have looked specifically at the effects of exercise in terms of helping stroke victims to recover, but much of this research can also be applied to other balance issues.

A study done in 2021 has indicated that balance can be improved quickly through exercise, and just a single session can make a significant difference to the individual's ability to balance. (2) The same study indicated that multiple sessions didn't offer much more benefit, but further research is needed to better understand this.

---

(1) Shephard, R.J. (1998). Aging and Exercise. In: Encyclopedia of Sports Medicine and Science, T.D.Fahey (Editor). Internet Society for Sport Science: http://sportsci.org. 7 March 1998. [Accessed: 13 May 2023]

(2) Leila Alizadehsaravi a b et al. (2021) The underlying mechanisms of improved balance after one and ten sessions of balance training in older adults, Human Movement Science. Available at:

https://www.sciencedirect.com/science/article/pii/S0167945721001585 [Accessed: 13 May 2023]

"in patients who performed physical exercise, there was a statistically significant decrease in both the number of falls and fallers." This tells us how important it is to use exercise when it comes to combatting balance problems.

How Does Exercise Help?

If you look at balance from a purely logical perspective, it makes sense that exercise would be key to improving it. After all, when you are standing upright, you are using a lot of muscles to keep yourself on your feet – and if those muscles are weak, you're much more likely to fall over. You may not feel like you're using muscles because the process is so automatic, but strengthening these muscles can give you more safety on your feet.

The stronger and better toned your muscles are, the more likely they are to be able to keep you upright, because they'll have more strength available to do so.

However, there's more to it than that. In order for these muscles to do their job, they need to be taking signals from the brain, which is telling them exactly how to balance. Your brain is, in turn, communicating with your eyes, ears, and the sensors in your legs, which give it information about your position relative to the ground.

When you practise balancing and perform exercises that challenge it, you encourage all of these things to work better, training both the muscles and the communication between the different parts. This twofold approach can make your balance significantly better in quite a short space of time.
If you're interested in learning more about how your balance fundamentally works, a lot of it relates to the inner ear – which might surprise you! Why the ear?

----

(3) Papalia, G. F., Papalia, R., Diaz Balzani, L. A., Torre, G., Zampogna, B., Vasta, S., Fossati, C., Alifano, A. M., & Denaro, V. (2020). The Effects of Physical Exercise on Balance and Prevention of Falls in Older People: A Systematic Review and Meta-Analysis. Journal of clinical medicine, 9(8), 2595. [Accessed: 13 May 2023]

The inner ear contains the vestibular system, which is made up of a complex maze of bone and soft tissue. The system contains structures called semicircular canals, and these have three ducts filled with fluids. These ducts form loops that are at approximate right angles to each other.

Each of the ducts has a structure at one end, called a cupula. This is a stretchy structure, and it is surrounded by a group of sensory hair cells. These have thin extensions that stick into the cupula, known as stereocilia.

When you turn your head, the fluid inside the canal flows towards or away from the cupulae, and this causes the cupulae to flex, bending the stereocilia. This stimulates a signal to the brain, which tells you which way you have turned your head. That helps you to figure out where your body is in relation to the ground, and tells your muscles what to do to keep you upright.

Hopefully, that has given you a little bit more of an understanding about how the different parts of your body work together to create balance. Remember, though, that while the inner ear contains the mechanism necessary for allowing you to balance, it's your muscles that do most of the work – and they're the part that you have control over.

That's why we're going to plunge into assessing your balance levels next, and then move on to looking at how you can improve your stability through exercise!

How to assess your current stability and balance levels

You might feel unsure about how much improvement your balance needs – and whether you actually need to work on it. In this section, we're going to cover a few simple ways you can test your balance at home.

1-Leg Balance Test

This is the easiest sort of test to perform by yourself at home. You should select a spot where you can stand on a flat surface, preferably with a wall or a stable chair nearby so you can place a hand on it if necessary. Ideally, you should also have a visible clock so you can check how long you can balance for.

Stand up straight, and then lift one of your feet off the floor, so you are standing on one leg. Keep your hands at your sides, or lift them out if that makes it easier.

Test how long you are able to balance for. If it is less than 30 seconds, you need to work on your balance. If you can stand up like this for over a minute, your balance is good, although it never hurts to improve it! Many adults find that they can easily manage a minute or more when they are young, but this starts to drop as they age.

2-Balancing On Both Feet

For this exercise, stand on a flat, stable surface, and place your feet together, so that your ankle bones are touching. Cross your arms over your chest, and close your eyes.

Stay as still as you can. When you feel yourself losing your balance, open your eyes and check the clock. Again, less than 30 seconds indicates that there is a problem, while more than a minute indicates that your balance is good.

3-Balancing On The Ball Of Your Foot

Again, choose a flat, stable surface, with a wall nearby so you can touch it if you need support.

Place your hands on your hips and lift one leg off the floor. Place that foot against the inside knee of your supporting leg.

Next, lift the heel of your supporting leg off the floor, so you are standing in the ball of your foot. Hold this position for as long as you can.

With each of these exercises, it's a good idea to test on both legs, to see if one leg is better than the other. You should then have a sense of how good your balance is – and whether that leaves you with an increased sense of confidence or feeling keen to improve, let's look next at how to figure out where your areas of weakness are.

Identifying areas of weakness and imbalance & how to quickly improve them

The first thing to do if you're struggling with your balance is to speak to your doctor to rule out any medical causes. If your balance issues are the result of medication, it's possible that your doctor can adjust the doses or provide something else to help. If you have an ear infection or another physical ailment, they may be able to offer treatment.

A doctor can also provide you with some balance tests, including a rotary chair, a video head impulse test, a dynamic visual acuity test, and videonystagmography, among others. These may help to identify issues with the inner ear and the eye muscles, which can be difficult to diagnose at home. Always take the time to speak to a physician before you start trying to improve your balance.

However, you can also spend time thinking about how you feel when balancing. A lot of different muscle groups are working to hold you upright, and you may find it useful to consider these, and to weigh up whether any in particular feel weak.

For example, if you notice that your ankles are shaking or hurting while you're balancing, it's likely that the muscles aren't strong enough there. If you find that your abdomen is straining and uncomfortable, this could indicate that you need to work on your core.

Start by making an effort to strengthen the muscles in that particular area. If you already work out frequently, you can easily build this into your routine. Doing just 5 minutes of ankle exercises per day could give you the strength you need to feel safer on your feet. Alternatively, training your core muscles may be the answer.

We're going to look in more detail at the exercises you can do later in this book – but at the centre of good balance is consistent practise. Make practising a regular part of your day, and you will soon see improvements.

For example, you might spend a few minutes balancing before or after brushing your teeth, or just before getting into bed. You can also practise as part of your exercise routine if you regularly exercise. The best way to quickly improve your balance is to make a point of challenging your muscles and your body's communication system as frequently as possible.

You should soon see improvements if you do this. Remember that like any kind of physical training, regular work is necessary, and you need to commit.

Next, we're going to look at some of the dangers associated with poor balance, and what you can do to prevent these.

Dangers of lack of stability
& how to prevent them for good

Being poorly balanced has some very clear, inherent dangers.

The dangers of lack of stability can be divided up into two categories: physical and mental. The two link together closely.

The Physical Dangers

The physical dangers are particularly obvious. Poor balance accounts for a large number of falls, especially among seniors. This can lead to a wide range of injuries, some as minor as bruising, and others as major as broken bones or even death. Falls can be dangerous anywhere, whether you're at home or out and about.

They are particularly problematic for the elderly, who may have poor bone health and often heal more slowly, but even young people can be badly injured or killed by a fall. Falls can exacerbate other conditions, and may result in lengthy hospital stays and loss of mobility.

Falls on stairs are the biggest danger for many people. Bear this in mind if you live in a two-storey home, and take appropriate precautions to protect yourself.

The Mental Problems

In terms of the mental impact, poor balance is also dangerous. Having a fall can destroy your confidence, but even just being constantly afraid of falling can do the same. You may feel that you can't go out and do things you would otherwise enjoy, and as a result, your quality of life may be reduced.

In terms of the mental impact, poor balance is also dangerous. Having a fall can destroy your confidence, but even just being constantly afraid of falling can do the same. You may feel that you can't go out and do things you would otherwise enjoy, and as a result, your quality of life may be reduced.

Some people find that their overall sense of well-being also deteriorates. Not feeling safe on your feet leads to low mood and unhappiness, and often triggers a sense of insecurity that can be surprisingly deeply rooted. You might feel upset and resentful if you have to depend on others for things you used to do yourself, and you may become hyper-aware of your age and the difficulties you face.

Loss of balance may not sound like a big deal on the surface, but it will impact almost every aspect of your life, and it shouldn't be underestimated.

The physical and mental impacts combined often result in individuals giving up activities that are important to them, because they feel unsafe doing them. This can even exacerbate the balance issues, because if you decrease your activities and don't challenge yourself, you'll find your muscles weaken and you are even less capable of balancing.

Of course, you don't want to be performing activities that are no longer safe for you, but you also don't want to just give up and accept that this is how life is now. There are things you can do to empower yourself and regain your confidence and capability.

That's why it's so important to combat balance issues effectively, and not to just ignore it if you feel you are less stable on your feet than you used to be. You'll increase your sense of independence, allow yourself to enjoy more activities, and improve your overall well-being, while reducing your risk of potentially serious injuries.

4 BIGGEST MISTAKES SENIORS MAKE THAT PREVENT THEM FROM BEING MORE STABLE ON THEIR FEET

It's important for seniors to recognise that as we age, the way we stand and move changes. When young adults walk around, the power necessary for movement is evenly distributed across 3 areas: the hips, the knees, and the ankles. These areas each account for about 1/3rd of your movement at this age. Your weight is spread across them, and they work to keep you stable and upright.

However, when you get a little older, your hips begin providing a lot more of the power – up to 75 percent in most senior adults. The visible differences may be subtle, but it changes how your body is working and how you are balancing in some significant ways. Your knees and ankles are doing a lot less work, and you may feel less stable as a result.

That's why it's really important to adjust how you approach movement, and to avoid making mistakes based on how your body used to behave.

MISTAKE 1) FAILURE TO EXERCISE

As you age, your muscles tend to get weaker and less capable of supporting your body weight. You may also become less active, because you might stop working, and you may spend more time relaxing (e.g. after retirement). A lot of seniors don't make the effort to keep themselves in good shape, and this can lead to balance problems.

You might think that your muscle strength doesn't have a lot to do with balance if it's your inner ear that's responsible for this – but you're using hundreds of muscles when you stand up, and even when you're motionless, you're still engaging a lot of muscles to keep yourself upright. Your quads, your glutes, your calves, your hamstrings, and your core muscles may all be working.

Some of these muscles are hard to exercise, and that means you need to put even more effort into making sure that they stay toned and have the strength to support your body.

It may be tempting to slow down and take it easy as you head into your senior years, but continuing to exercise is crucial. No matter what you decide to do as part of your exercise routine, make sure you keep your body moving, and don't let your muscles waste. You should aim to do some exercise every day, with the occasional rest day, to keep your body in good condition.

If you have health conditions that make exercising difficult or you're not sure about it, you may want to talk to a doctor or a physiotherapist about your current physical condition and what exercises you can do safely. They should be able to provide guidance and resources that will allow you stay in shape.

Mistake 2) Wearing The Wrong Shoes

Your shoes make a massive difference to how well balanced you are, and can really affect your stability. A lot of shoes simply lack the support that you might need to stay balanced. Many seniors opt for comfortable slippers, especially if laces have become challenging, but you shouldn't just grab the first pair of slip-on shoes you can find. They could be dangerous and undermine your stability.

If you're not feeling very safe on your feet anymore, it's often a good idea to look at shoes that have been specifically designed for athletes. These tend to offer more support, and will often have non-slip soles designed to prevent falls.

Getting some that fit you very well is also important. You can go to a store and ask them for help with the fitting, and you'll probably find you feel much more stable when you have your shoes on.

Avoid shoes that are backless or loose, as these very frequently contribute to fall risks, and can make you feel less stable and safe. Soft soles or shoes that are very worn out can also be problematic. Opt for shoes in good condition, that fit comfortably and are snug on your feet.

MISTAKE 3) NOT BEING SELF-AWARE

It can be hard to adjust when you've gone from being fit, healthy, and well-balanced. You might try to do things exactly as you used to, without thinking about how your physical abilities may have changed. You may not pay much attention to how you move stand, bend, reach, lean, and turn.

This leads to an increased risk of falls, and reduces your stability. You need to get into the habit of thinking about how you move, especially if you need to bend over to pick something up, or lean forwards to tie your shoes.

Practising self-awareness takes time, but it's very manageable. Try to pause before you move, and think about what the movement will involve. Sometimes, just being aware in this way can make you better able to balance, because you'll be thinking about how your limbs are positioned.

You may find that it helps to tie a ribbon around your finger or something similar while you are practising self-awareness. This can remind you to think about it, keeping it at the forefront of your mind and preventing you from forgetting. It probably won't offer a foolproof solution, but it can certainly help.

MISTAKE 4) NOT CHALLENGING YOURSELF

Although you do need to be careful and take the right approach to balance, it's good to challenge yourself – in the correct environment. You want your balance to improve, not just stagnate, and that often involves pushing just a little beyond your comfort zone.

Try to find moments in which you can challenge yourself, while maintaining your safety. For example, consider testing your balance on a firm but soft surface (such as a cork mat) and make sure you have a way to call for help if you need it.

Do keep challenging yourself, though, even if you feel unsure about doing so. While it's important to feel safe and to respect your limits, you should make sure you are taking steps to improve your balance whenever you have an opportunity. If you don't, you're likely to find that it gets worse over time, and it's harder to improve.

In some cases, challenging yourself might involve attending a fitness class or something similar. For example, you could consider a yoga or tai chi class. They can be combined with the exercises in this book to ensure you're making progress and things are improving.

If you avoid those four mistakes, you should find that you stay in pretty good shape in your senior years, and this can really help with your balance and coordination. With that in mind, let's cover some aspects of diet that can also help, and then we'll move on to exercises!

Food & supplements recommended by experts for improved balance & stability

It's easy to forget the importance of diet when it comes to physical conditions like instability, but what you eat and the nutrients you give to your body can be of crucial importance too. There are quite a few nutrients that affect balance, so let's cover a few of them.

Take Vitamin D

The National Institutes Of Health recommends taking vitamin D supplements, for several reasons. One is that vitamin D is necessary for the development of muscle fibres, and not having enough vitamin D can lead to pain and muscle weakness. It's thought that as many as 1 in 6 adults in the UK could be deficient in vitamin D.

You can get vitamin D in tablet form, but spending time outside is also key to getting enough vitamin D. If you live in the UK, you will probably want to do both, as the sun is only strong enough for us to produce sufficient amounts of vitamin D from April to September. Throughout the rest of the year, supplements are important for making sure you get enough vitamin D.

You can also get vitamin D from your food, from things like oily fish, liver, red meat, and egg yolkst. It's also found in some plant milks and spreads, as well as breakfast cereals.

Eat Dark-Skinned Fruits

Another study, presented by the lead researcher Jane Cavanaugh, indicated that dark-skinned fruits, such as blueberries and grapes, can be very beneficial for balance, as reported by SaveOurBones. The reason for this is that they contain something called resveratrol, which improves your balance and your coordination.

It's thought that you are best taking resveratrol in via food, which is why it's important to eat some of these fruits if you can. Foods that contain resveratrol include bilberries, red grapes, blueberries, cranberries, and peanuts.

---

(5) Department of Health and Social Care. (2022). Retrieved from

https://www.gov.uk/government/news/new-review-launched-into-vitamin-d-intake-to-help-tackle-health-disparities

[Accessed: May 15 2023]

(6) Vivian Goldschmidt, M. (2016). Retrieved from https://saveourbones.com/5-foods-that-improve-balance/

[Accessed: May 15 2023]

TAKE VITAMIN B12

Vitamin B12 may have some impact on stability too. Being deficient in vitamin B12 has a negative effect on your central nervous system, which can cause a whole host of other difficulties – and has a serious effect on your balance. A lot of studies have looked at this relationship, and if you have a vitamin B12 deficiency, your balance may suffer as a result.

Vitamin B12 is mostly found in animal products, so it's an area you're more likely to struggle with if you are vegan or vegetarian. You may want to get supplements to make sure you are getting everything you need from your diet.

It's always a good idea to eat a wide range of foods, so that you're taking in a good variety of vitamins and minerals. If you have any concerns about deficiencies, talk to your doctor. They may be able to do blood tests to check for deficiencies, and recommend supplements that will help you.

---

(7) Kul, Ayhan & BİLGE, Nuray & UZKESER, Hülya & SARIHAN, Köksal & Melikoglu, Meltem & BAYGUTALP, Fatih. (2020). Postural Stability and Risk of Fall in Vitamin B12 Deficiency. Fiziksel Tıp ve Rehabilitasyon Bilimleri Dergisi. 23. 144-151. 10.31609/jpmrs.2019-72113.

STEP BY STEP STATIC BALANCE EXERCISES FOR IMPROVED POSTURE & BALANCE

First, let's briefly cover what a static exercise is. Static exercises are those that involve keeping still in a certain position for a set period – usually up to 45 seconds. You might be standing, sitting, or lying down, depending on the pose. This can help to stretch your muscles, and may be a good place to start if you are lacking in confidence and you're afraid of falling.

With that in mind, let's look at some static exercises you can try! Remember that regardless of which exercises you going to attempt, you should choose a space where you feel safe, with a firm, comfortable surface under your feet. If you are not confident, consider exercising beside a chair or a wall, so you can easily put your hand on something to keep yourself upright.

EXERCISE 1
STILL STANDING

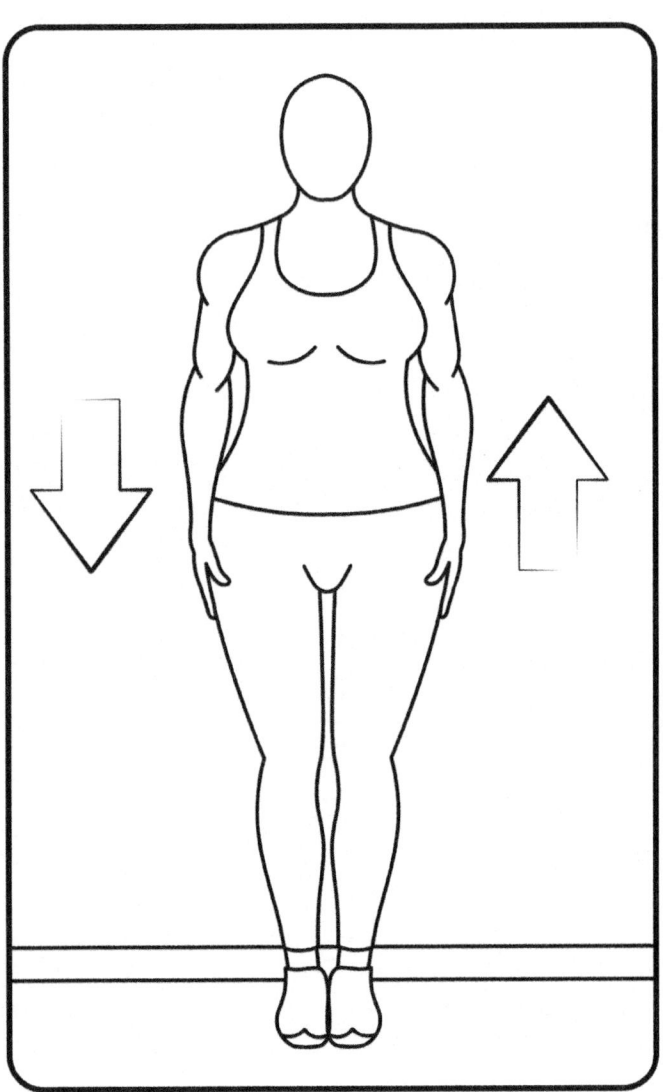

1.) On a flat surface, get into a basic standing position, with your arms at your sides and your feet about hip-width apart.

2.) Move your feet so that they are together underneath your body, with your ankle bones touching.

3.) Stand upright, looking straight ahead of you.

4.) Close your eyes and hold this position for 30 seconds.

5.) Relax.

EXERCISE 2
FOOT FORWARD

1.) On a flat surface, get into a basic standing position, with your arms at your sides.

2.) Step your right forward in front of your left one, so that your right foot's heel is close to your left foot's toes. You can adjust until you feel safe and comfortable, but try to keep your feet fairly close together.

3.) Hold this position for 30 seconds.

4.) Swap to the other side, and repeat this exercise with your left foot in front of your right foot.

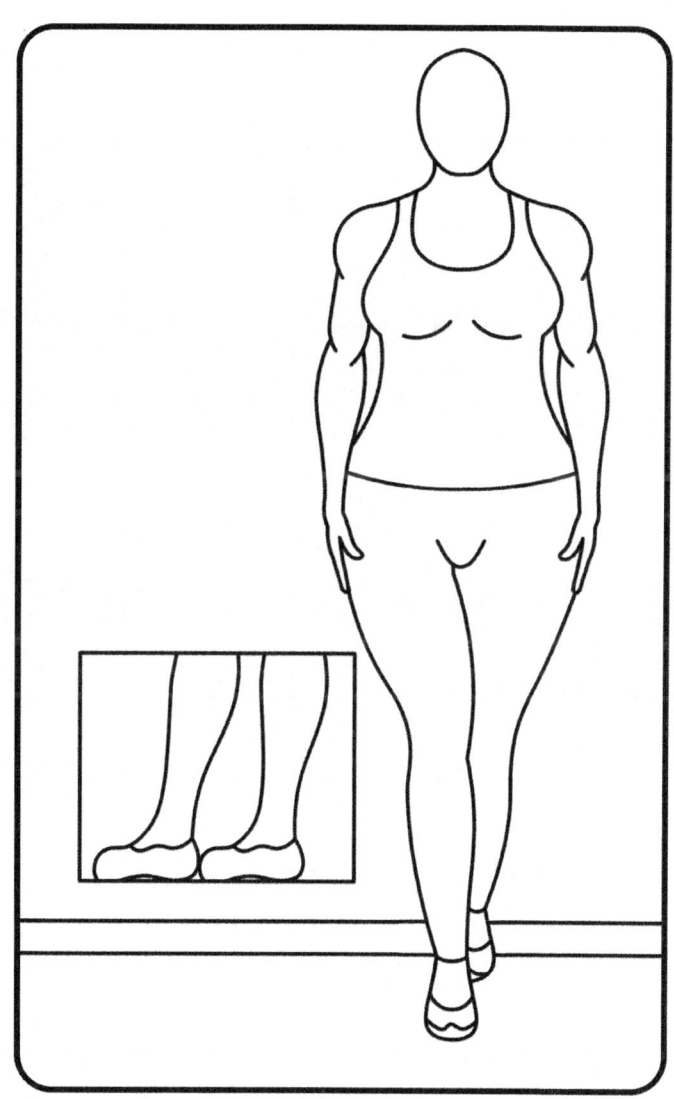

EXERCISE 3
BALANCING ON ONE FOOT

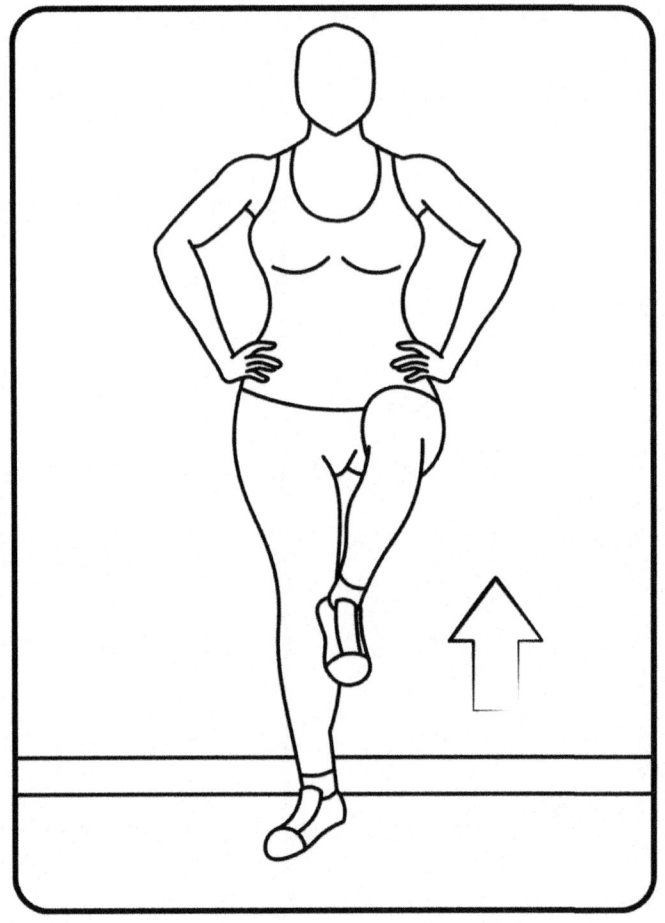

1.) Start on a flat surface in a basic standing position.

2.) Lift your right foot up from the floor to a point that feels comfortable and stable.

3.) Hold this position for 30 seconds.

4.) Put your right foot back on the floor, and swap so that your left foot is lifted up.

5.) Hold this position for 30 seconds.

EXERCISE 4
LIFTED FOOT BALANCE

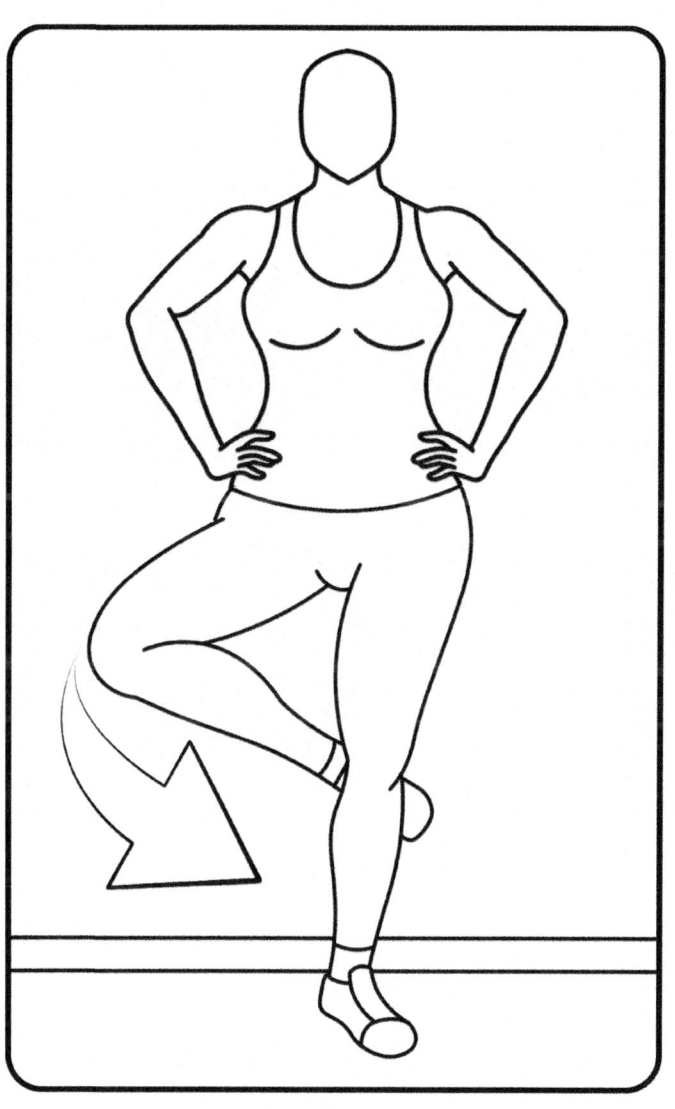

1.) Stand comfortably, and then lift your right foot from the floor and place the sole of your foot against the inside of your left knee.

2.) Hold this position for 45 seconds if you can.

3.) Lower your right foot back to the floor and then swap for the left foot and repeat the exercise.

EXERCISE 5
FOOT KICKED FORWARDS

1.) Stand comfortably, and then lift your right foot up in front of you, making sure you keep your body upright. Don't lean backwards or forwards.

2.) Lift your foot up carefully to an inch or two off the ground.

3.) Hold this position for 30 seconds.

4.) Lower your right foot back onto the floor.

5.) Lift your left foot a couple of inches off the ground in front of you.

6.) Hold this position for 30 seconds.

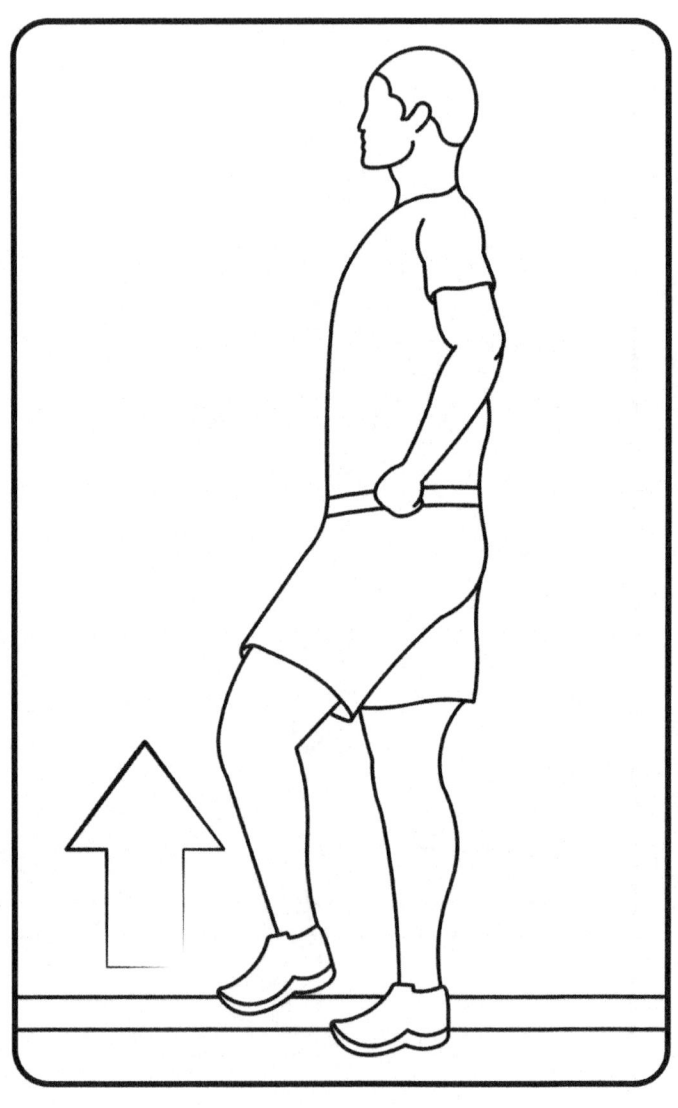

26

EXERCISE 6
FOOT KICKED BACK

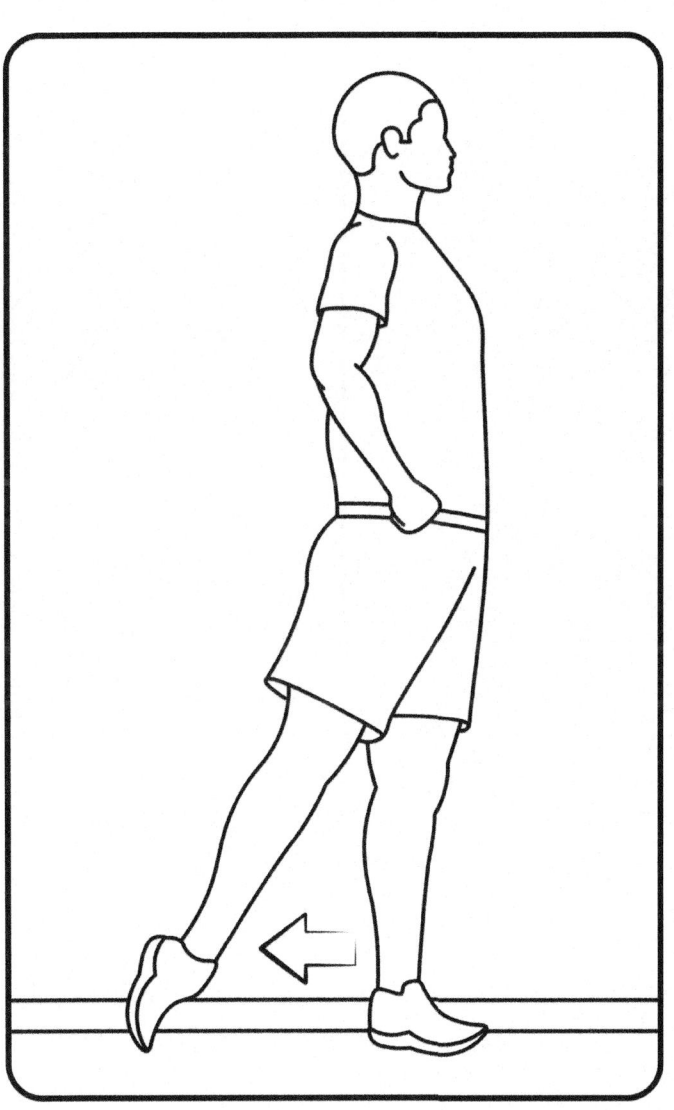

1.) Stand up straight, with your feet underneath your shoulders.

2.) Lift your right foot up and carefully pull it back behind you, so that your toes rest against your floor and the sole of your foot faces away from your body.

3.) Hold this position for 30 seconds.

4.) Place your right foot back under your body, and kick your left foot back.

5.) Hold this position for 30 seconds.

6.) Return to a standing position and relax.

EXERCISE 7
SIDE LEANS

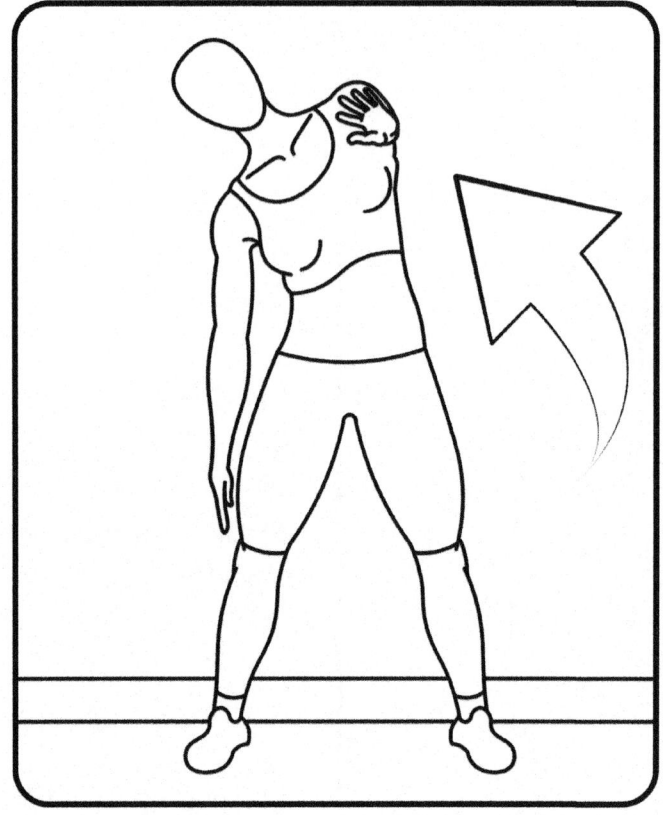

1.) Stand upright, with your feet underneath your hips and your arms relaxed by your sides.

2.) Lift your arms up to your body, and then reach your right arm out to the right, leaning your body carefully out too. Only move as far as feels comfortable for you. Make sure you stay steady as you move; don't tip forwards or backwards.

3.) Hold the position for several seconds, and then gradually bring your arms back into the centre and shift your body weight into the centre too.

4.) Move your left arm out to the left, and lean your body to the left as well. Again, keep your body from tipping forwards or backwards, or you may fall.

5.) Come back to the central position, and then repeat the movement twice on each side.

EXERCISE 8
BEANBAG BALANCE

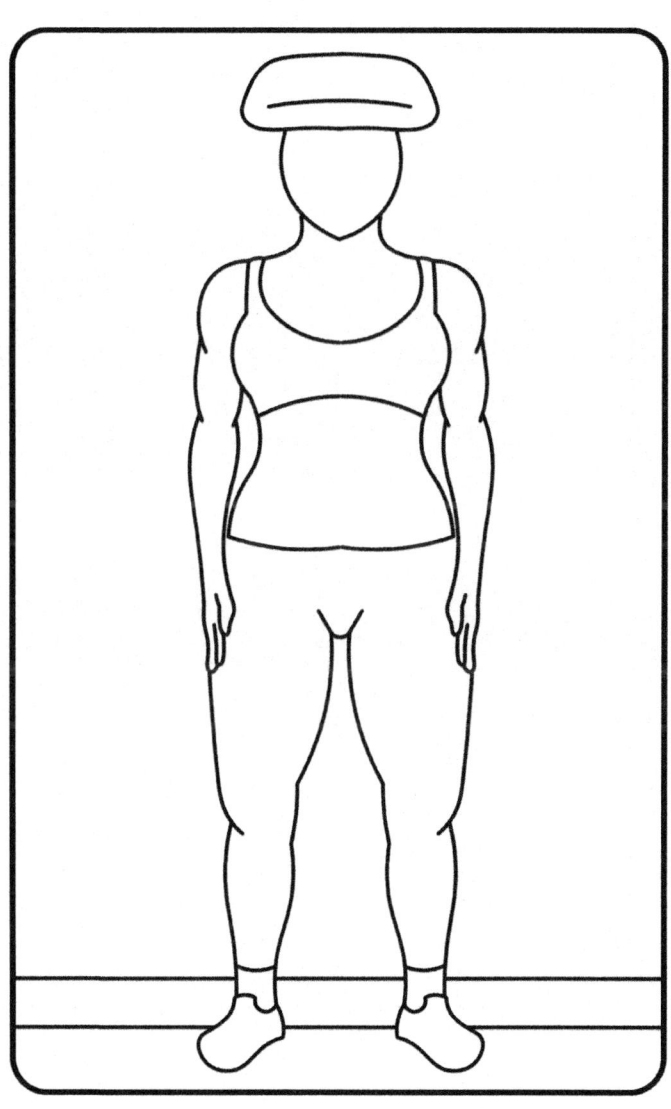

Note: For this exercise, you will need a beanbag or another small, soft, lightweight item you can place on your head. It needs to be heavy enough to slide off if you move, but not uncomfortable.

1.) Stand in an upright position, with your feet hip-width apart.

2.) Place the beanbag on your head and balance it there comfortably.

3.) Stand as still as you can. Pay attention to the muscles in your back and shoulders, and make sure you are as upright as you can be.

You may also find it useful to use the beanbag exercise when you are walking around your home. It can make you more aware of how you are standing and moving. Be careful if you need to pick it up, however; don't fall over.

EXERCISE 9
HEAD TURNING BALANCE

Note: Remember, your head is responsible for a lot of your ability to balance. Moving your head around can quickly throw your sense of balance, even if you felt stable before. This exercise is very good for improving the communication between your brain and your muscles, but undertake it with caution. Move your head slowly, and use a chair for additional support if you don't feel safe on your feet.

1.) Stand on a firm surface with your feet together.

2.) Gradually tilt your head back until you are looking at the ceiling.

3.) Bring your head back to the centre, and then look down at your feet. Keep your body upright and don't lean forwards.

4.) Stand on a firm surface with your feet together.

5.) Gradually tilt your head back until you are looking at the ceiling.

6.) Bring your head back to the centre, and then look down at your feet. Keep your body upright and don't lean forwards.

7.) Stand on a firm surface with your feet together.

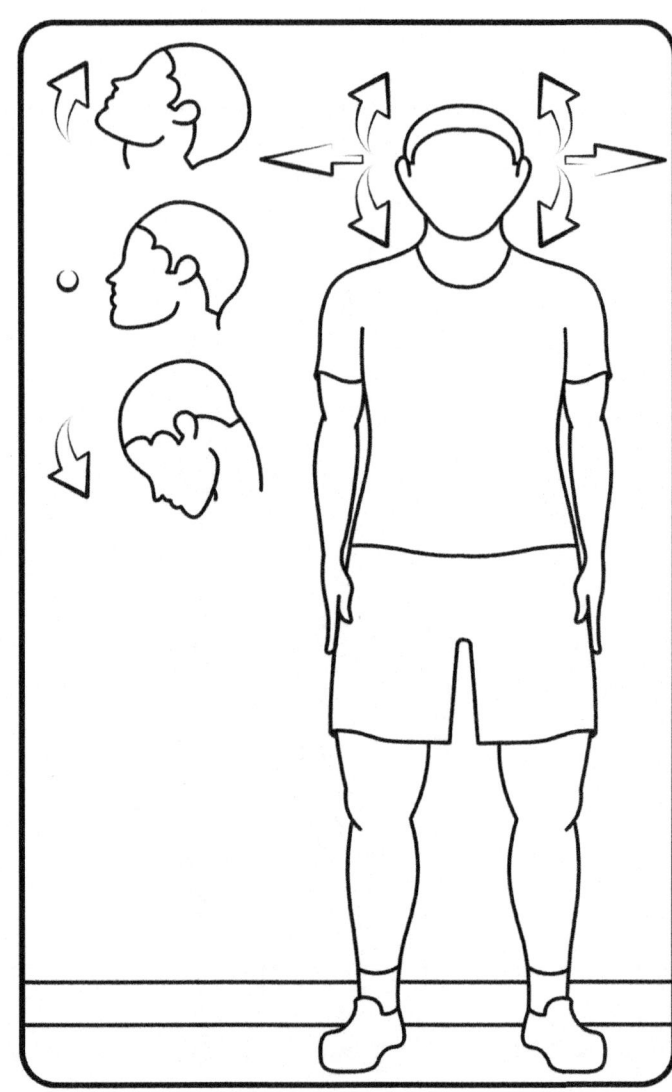

You may also find it useful to use the beanbag exercise when you are walking around your home. It can make you more aware of how you are standing and moving. Be careful if you need to pick it up, however; don't fall over.

STEP BY STEP DYNAMIC BALANCE EXERCISES FOR IMPROVED BALANCE & COORDINATION

Dynamic exercises are the opposite of static exercises: they involve movement while you are performing the exercise. Dynamic exercises can be a great way to hone your balance, because they involve moving your head around, which challenges the brain to keep track of how your body is relating to the floor. Dynamic exercises can be trickier, but a lot of people find them rewarding and beneficial.

With that in mind, let's check out some dynamic exercises you can do to improve your balance.

Exercise 1
Weight Shifting

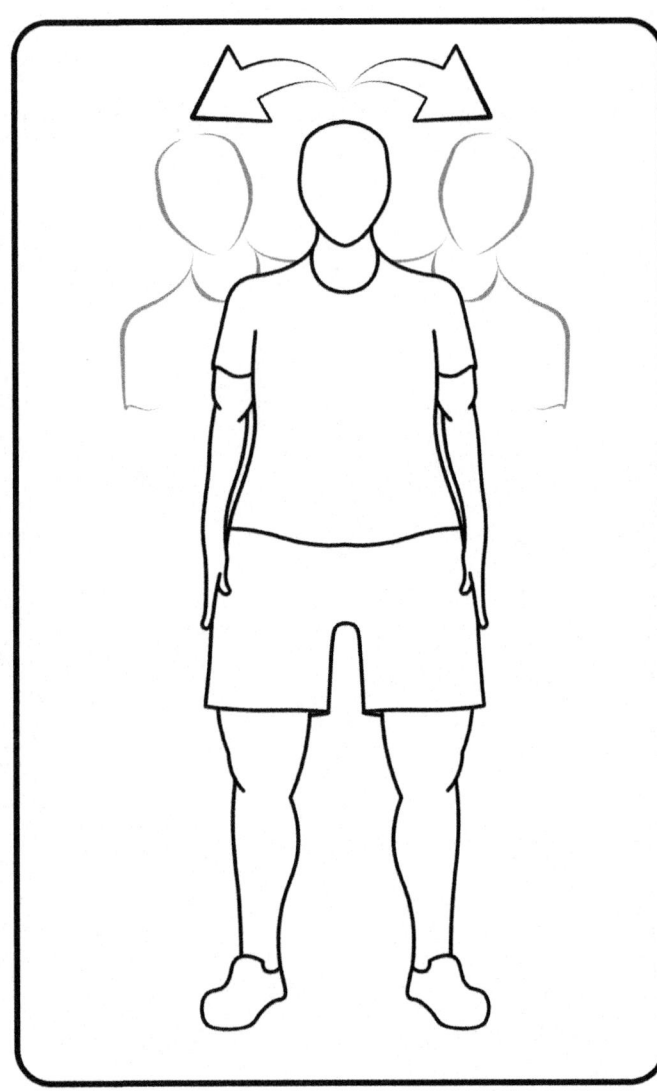

1.) Start in a basic standing position, with your body erect. Your feet should be slightly wider apart than your shoulders, and your weight should be evenly distributed throughout your body.

2.) Moving from your ankle upwards, start start shifting your weight from one side to the other, without taking your feet off the floor. Make sure you're moving your whole body, from ankle upwards, so your body stays in line with itself and you don't overbalance.

3.) Shift your weight gradually to the left, so your left leg is supporting your body, and then shift gradually to the right.

4.) Keep moving back and forth, making sure your whole body is moving, not just your hips.

5.) If you feel comfortable with this, gradually raise your left arm as you shift your body to the left, as though you were trying to reach for a high shelf. You can either look at your arm, or keep looking forwards as you move.

6.) Lower your left arm as you shift back to the central position, and then raise your right arm as you shift to the right.

7.) Continue this exercise for a couple of minutes, and then relax.

Exercise 2
Leg Curls

1.) Start in a basic standing position, and then lift and engage your chest.

2.) Lift your right foot off the floor and put it behind you, keeping your right knee close to your left knee.

3.) Lift your heel as high behind you as feels safe, and tense the muscles in your leg.

4.) Lower your right leg back to the floor, and shift your weight onto it.

5.) Lift your left foot off the floor and pull it up behind you, lifting it up as far as feels safe.

6.) Tense the muscles in your leg a few times, and then lower your foot back to the floor again.

7.) Repeat this exercise 3 times on either side.

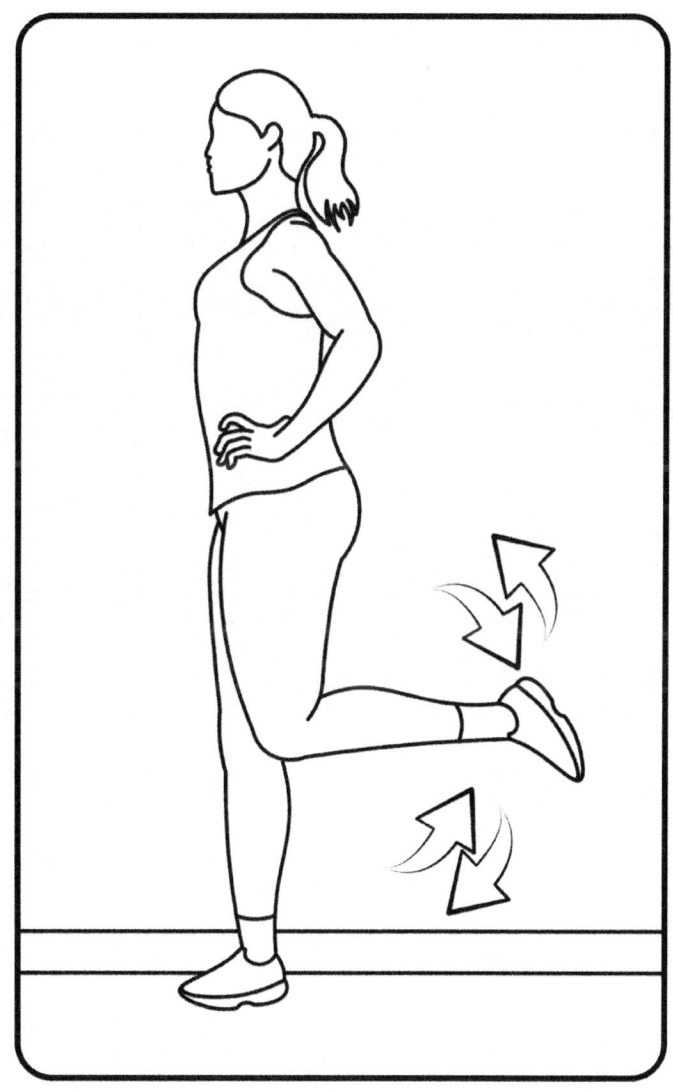

EXERCISE 3
TOE RISES

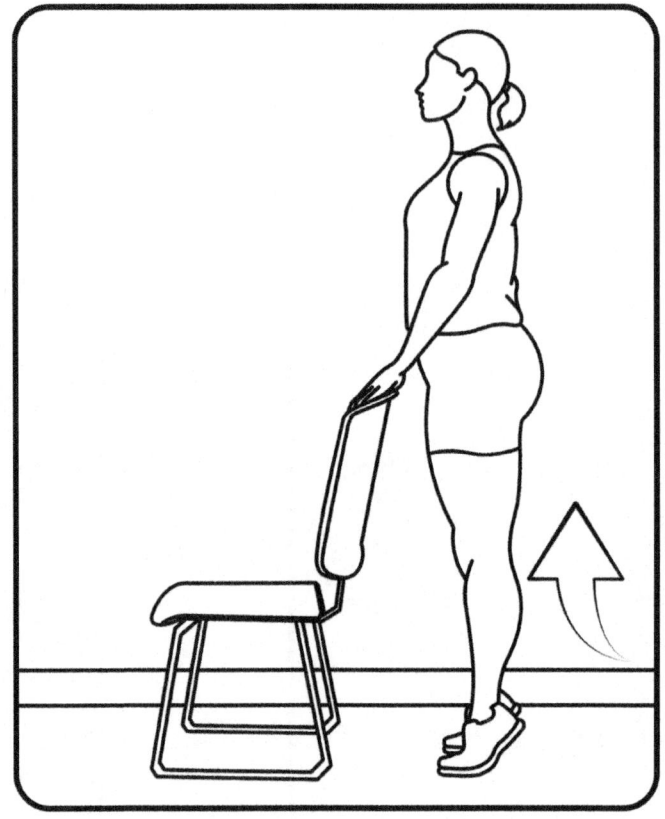

1.) Place a sturdy chair in front of you, so you are standing behind its back.

2.) Put your hands on the back of the chair, and then gradually rise up onto your toes. Stay there for the count of three.

3.) Lower yourself back onto the soles of your feet, in a controlled manner.

4.) Lift back up onto your toes, and again hold for three seconds.

5.) Lower back onto the soles of your feet. Keep repeating this for a couple of minutes, making sure your movements are controlled.

EXERCISE 4
KNEE LIFTS

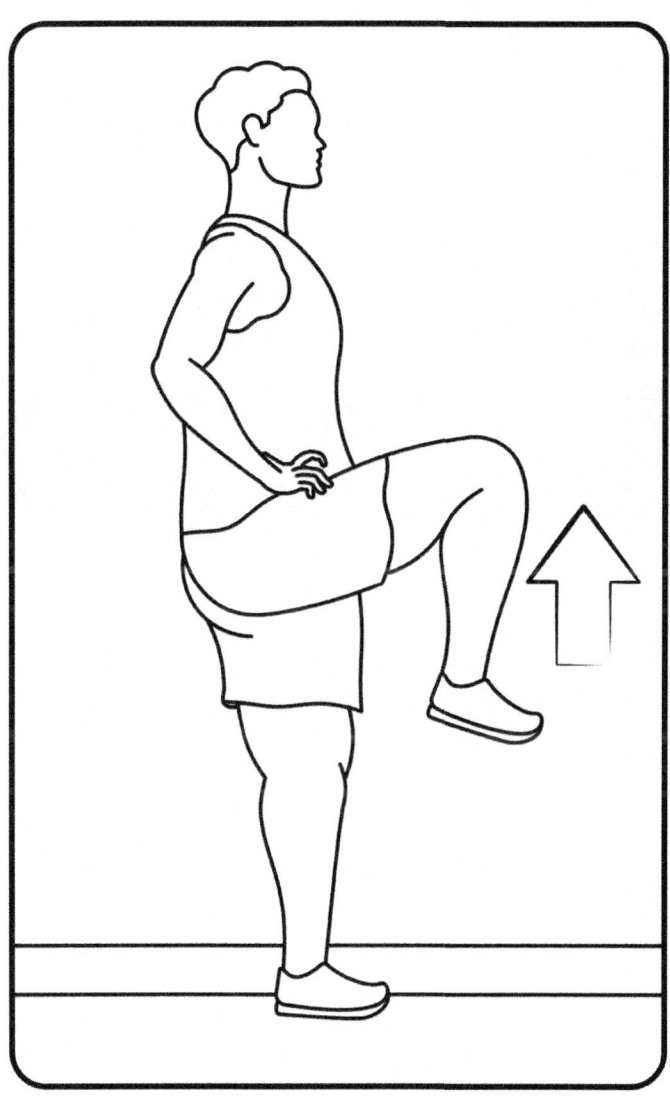

1.) Stand upright on a flat surface, with your weight evenly distributed between your legs, and your feet beneath your hips.

2.) Shift your weight onto your left leg, and lift your right knee up towards your chest as high as feels comfortable for you. Once you hit the top comfort position, hold it for a few seconds. You can hold onto your leg or knee with your hands if this makes things easier.

3.) In a controlled fashion, lower your foot back to the floor.

4.) Shift your weight onto your right leg, and lift your left knee up as high as you can.

5.) Keep repeating this for 3 cycles on each side, and then relax.

6.) You can make this exercise more challenging by performing it with your eyes closed.

Note that when you begin this exercise, you may need some support from either the wall or a chair. That's fine, but work towards not needing it, and only use it as much as you need in order to stay safe.

EXERCISE 5
SIDEWAYS WALKING

1.) Start in the central standing position, with your arms relaxed by your sides.

2.) Step your right foot out to the side until it is a bit further than your shoulder, moving in a controlled manner.

3.) Step your left foot out to the other side, again making sure you are in control.

4.) Step your right foot back into the central position, and then bring the left foot in again too.

5.) Repeat this 5 to 10 times, making sure you are in control at all times. Your torso should stay upright as you step.

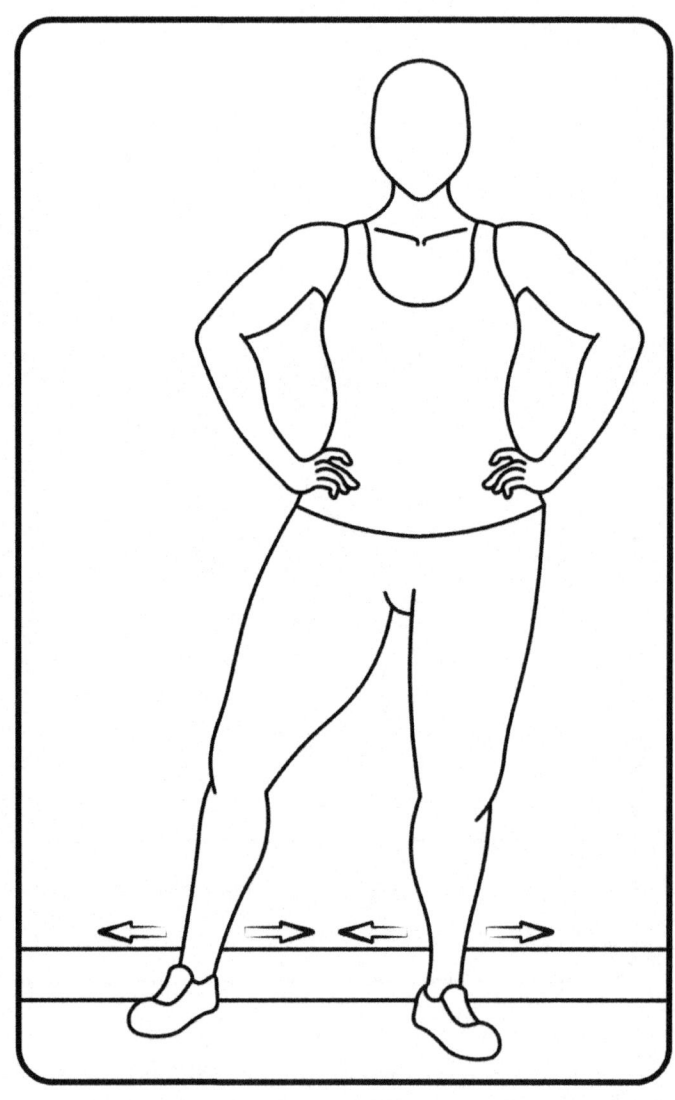

EXERCISE 6
CROSS-OVERS

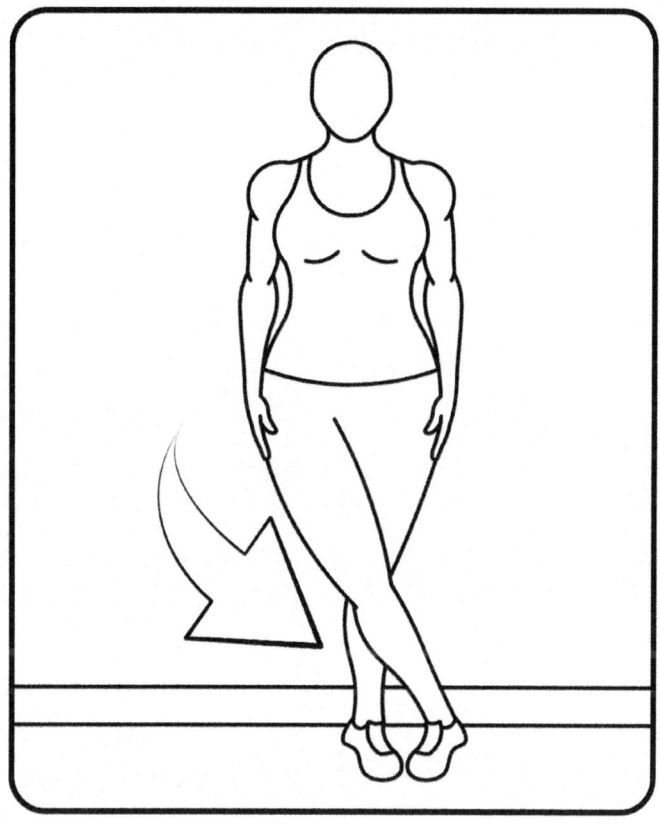

1.) Place a sturdy chair in front of you, so you are standing behind its back.

2.) Put your hands on the back of the chair, and then gradually rise up onto your toes. Stay there for the count of three.

3.) Lower yourself back onto the soles of your feet, in a controlled manner.

4.) Lift back up onto your toes, and again hold for three seconds.

5.) Lower back onto the soles of your feet. Keep repeating this for a couple of minutes, making sure your movements are controlled.

EXERCISE 7
WEIGHT SHIFTING

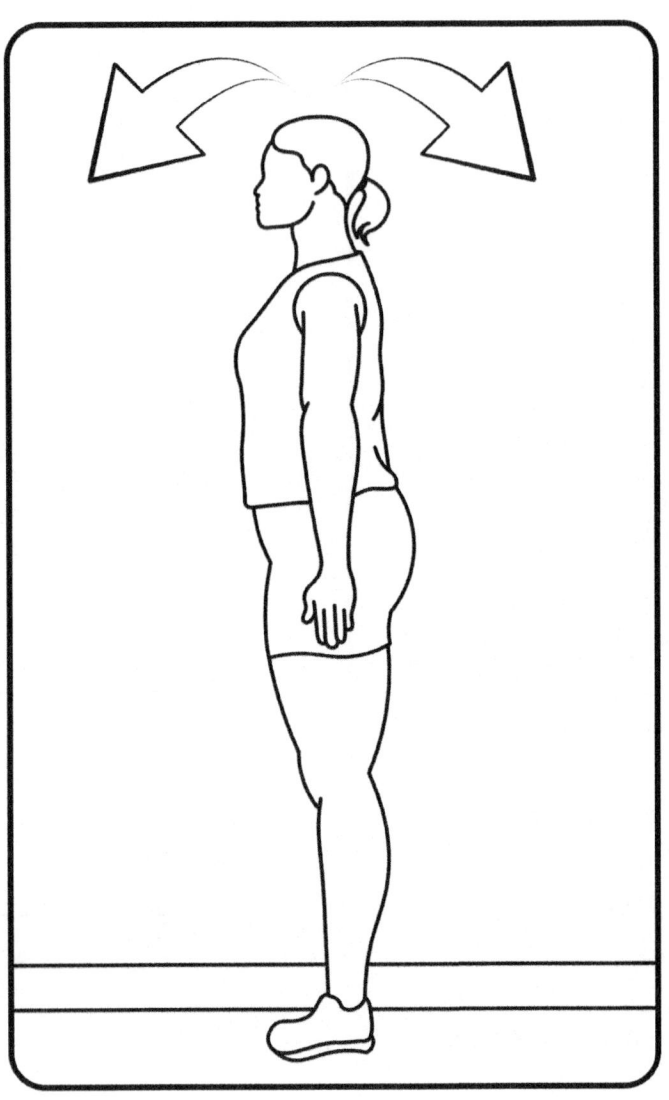

1.) Stand in a central position, with your feet hip-width apart and your arms resting by your sides. Your weight should be evenly distributed between your feet.

2.) Use your ankles to shift your weight from the centre to the front, and then to the back. You will need to stick your hips back a little way as you move backwards, or you may lose your balance.

3.) Keep shifting backwards and forwards, using your ankles to make sure your whole body is moving.

4.) Return your weight to the central position, and relax.

Exercise 8
Hip Abductions

1.) Stand with a chair nearby so you can put your hand on it for support if necessary.

2.) Stand upright, and then lift your right arm up and begin to lean gradually to the right.

3.) As you lean, pick your left foot up off the floor and move it out to your left.

4.) Hold this position for a few seconds, and then lower your left foot back to the floor and lower your right arm back to your side.

5.) Repeat this exercise by stretching out to the left with your left arm, and lifting your right foot a little way from the floor.

6.) Return to the central position, and repeat 3 times on each side.

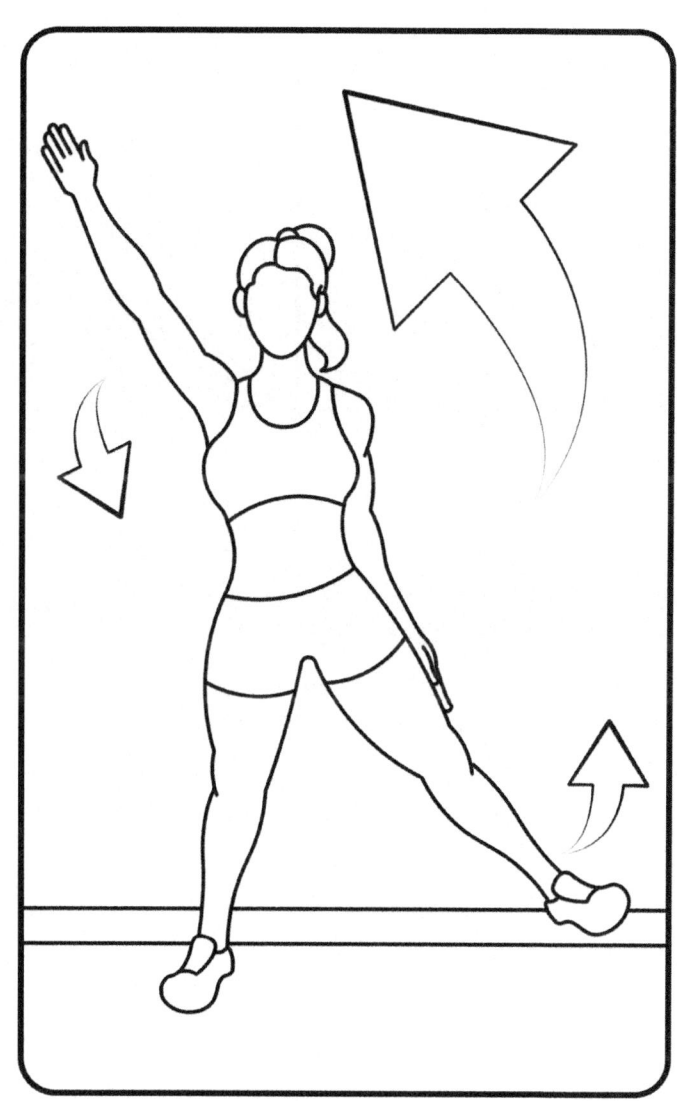

Exercise 9
Rocking The Boat

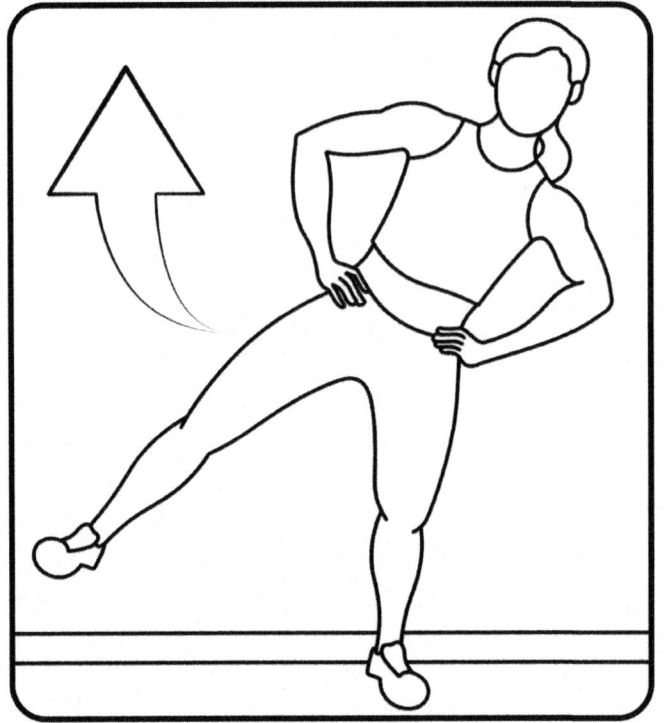

1.) Stand with your feet hip-width apart, and your body upright and straight.

2.) Press your weight down into your feet firmly, putting equal pressure on each foot.

3.) Shift your weight onto your left leg, and lift your right foot off the floor.

4.) Hold your right foot up for 30 seconds. You may wish to keep it still, or to roll your ankle. Stay as stable as you can.

5.) Lower your right foot back to the floor and shift your weight onto your right leg.

6.) Lift your left foot off the floor and repeat the exercise.

7.) Do this 5 times on each side.

EXERCISE 10
STEP AND BEND

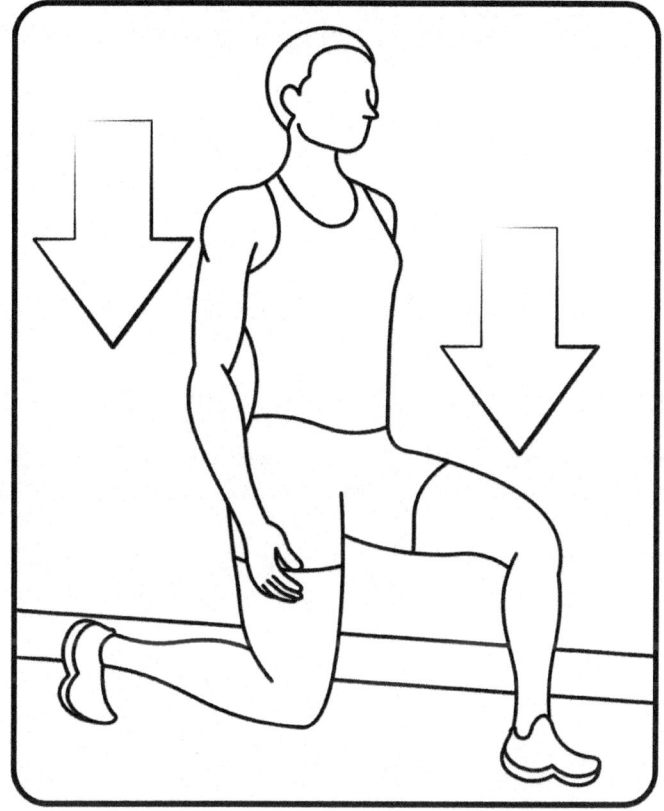

1.) Begin standing up straight, with your feet hip-width apart.

2.) Shift your weight onto your left leg, and step forwards with your right leg. Place your foot firmly on the floor.

3.) As you do so, bend your body forwards as though you were stooping to pick something up. Only go as far as feels comfortable, and then stop.

4.) Gradually, with control, come back up to the central position, with both feet under your body.

5.) Shift your weight onto your right leg and step forwards with your left leg, repeating the exercise on this side.

6.) Do this 5 times per side. If you would find it easier, have something you can reach for, such as a stool or chair you can pretend you are going to pick up.

Step by step proprioceptive exercises to enhance sensory awareness & balance control

In case you're not familiar with the term, proprioception is the sense that allows your brain to figure out how your body is moving, and how it relates to the rest of the world.

It pays attention to your body's actions, its location, and the movement that's going on. It's sometimes known as kinesthesia, and it involves a range of complicated sensations, including how you perceive the movement of your joints and their current position, and the force your muscles are exerting.

You use proprioception when you take note of how much force you are using, and when you assess the speed you're moving with, as well as the timing of your movements.

Proprioception is key to everyday life, and without it, you wouldn't be able to move your limbs in the external environment effectively. It's vital when you're exercising – so we're going to cover some exercises that are particularly good for proprioception. Let's get started!

EXERCISE 1
TABLE TOP

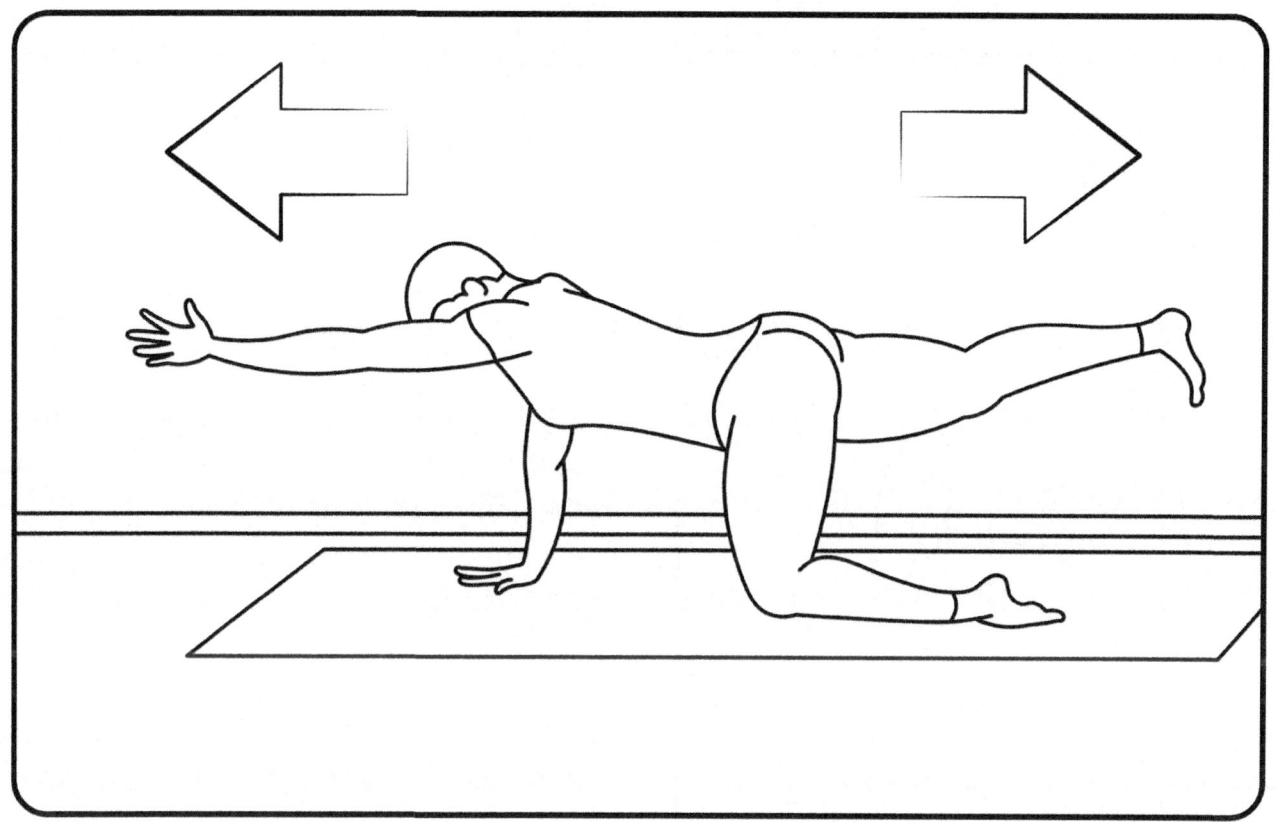

1.) Get on all fours, with your arms under your shoulders and your knees under your hips. Flatten your back and align your neck with your spine, so your back and neck are as straight as possible. You should be looking at the floor.

2.) Lift your right arm up and extend it out in front of you. At the same time, lift your left leg and extend it out behind you. Hold your core muscles tight.

3.) Hold this position for about 5 seconds, and then lower your arm and leg back to the floor.

4.) Repeat this on the other side. Repeat around 5 times on each side.

5.) If you are feeling confident and you would like to increase the challenge, close your eyes and hold the position for 10 seconds, rather than 5.

EXERCISE 2
WALKING CROSS

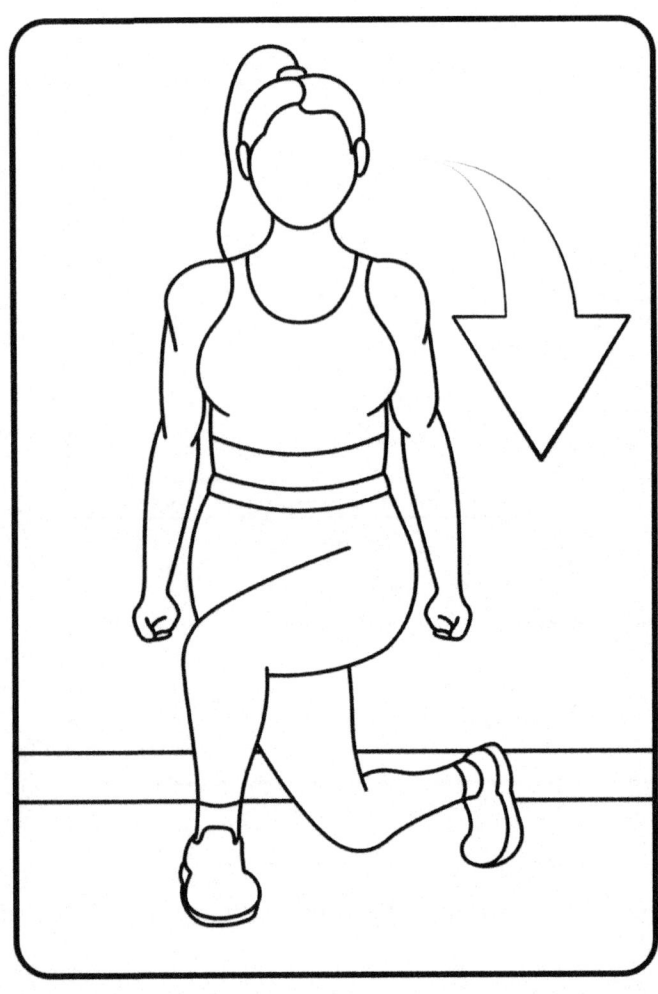

1.) Start near one side of the room, with a clear space on either side of you.

2.) Lift your left leg off the floor and bring your knee up as high as feels comfortable.

3.) Set your left foot on the far side of your right foot, so your legs are crossed. Try to twist your hips as you complete the motion.

4.) Uncross your legs by moving your right foot to the side of your left, so you are standing to the right of where you started.

5.) Again, lift your left leg off the floor, bring your knee up high, and then set your left foot on the far side of your right foot.

6.) Uncross your legs by moving your right foot to the side of your left, so you are once more in the normal standing position.

7.) Keep repeating this until you have moved several paces to the right.

8.) Begin to move to the left by raising your right knee up high, crossing it in front of your left leg, and placing your right foot on the far side of your left foot.

9.) As before, uncross your legs so that your left foot is back on the left, and continue the motion.

10.) Keep doing this until you are back where you started.

44

EXERCISE 3
SQUAT TO STAND

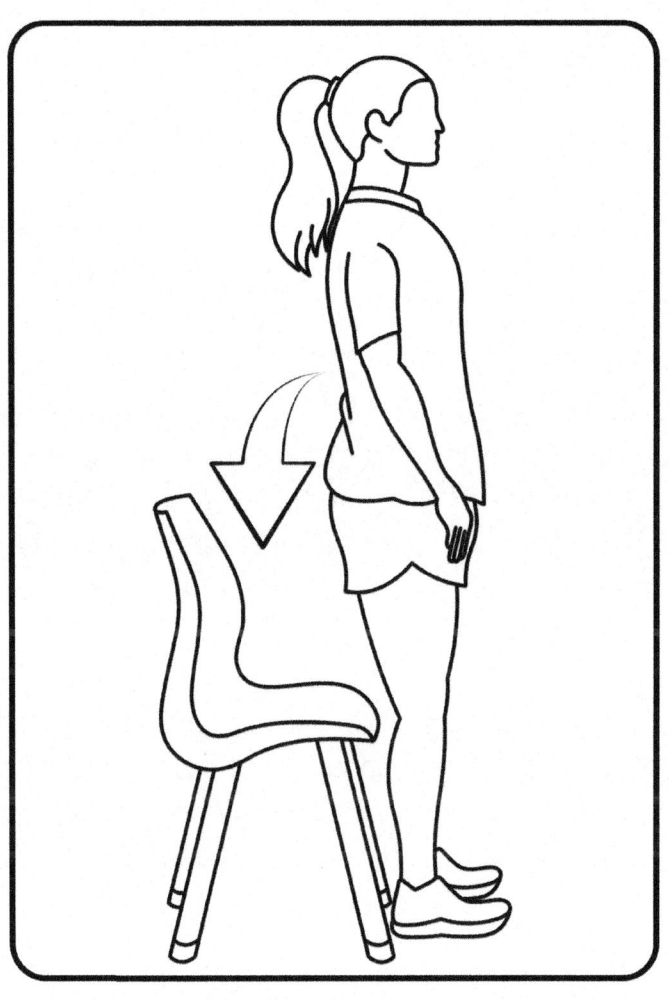

2.) Begin to engage your core muscles to lift yourself up from the chair, without using your hands to push yourself.

3.) Keep engaging your core and your legs, until you rise up from the chair and reach a standing position. Make sure you fully stand up; many people stop before they have completely straightened their backs, which decreases the value of the exercise.

4.) In a controlled manner, start to sit back down, moving gradually. Keep your core muscles engaged. You can hold your arms out in front of you to give yourself better balance if this helps.

5.) Sit back in the chair. It's okay if you initially drop the last few inches, but aim for control on the whole descent.

6.) Sit for a moment, and then stand up again.

7.) Do this 5 times if you are able to.

Note: you will need a sturdy chair on a non-slip surface for this exercise. Make sure it is stable before you begin the exercise, as you may find you need to drop back into it in a hurry if the exercise is too challenging for you initially.

1.) Sit comfortably in a chair, with your hands resting at your sides and your feet firmly planted on the floor.

Exercise 4
Squat Jump

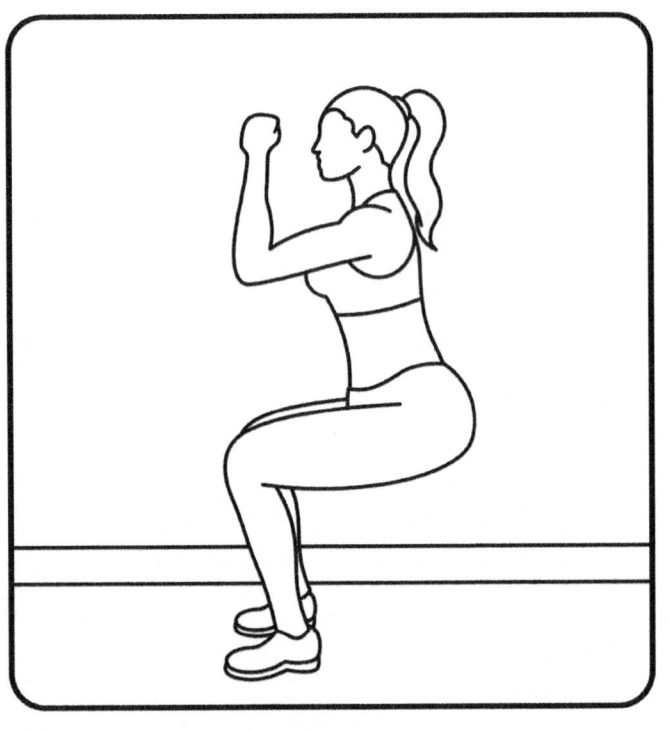

1.) Stand up very straight, with your feet shoulder-width apart and your knees slightly bent.

2.) Gradually squat down. The goal is to get your thighs parallel with the floor, but only go as far as you feel comfortable. You will feel your hips moving backwards. Keep your back straight and your head up. Your weight should be mostly on your heels.

3.) Hold the squat for a second, and then push yourself quickly upwards, reaching your arms into the air. You may feel safe to actually jump slightly, or you may wish to keep your feet on the floor. Either approach is fine.

4.) Drop back down into your squat, getting your thighs as close to parallel with the floor as you can manage.

5.) Swing your arms back up and jump again. Repeat this around 5 times if you are able to.

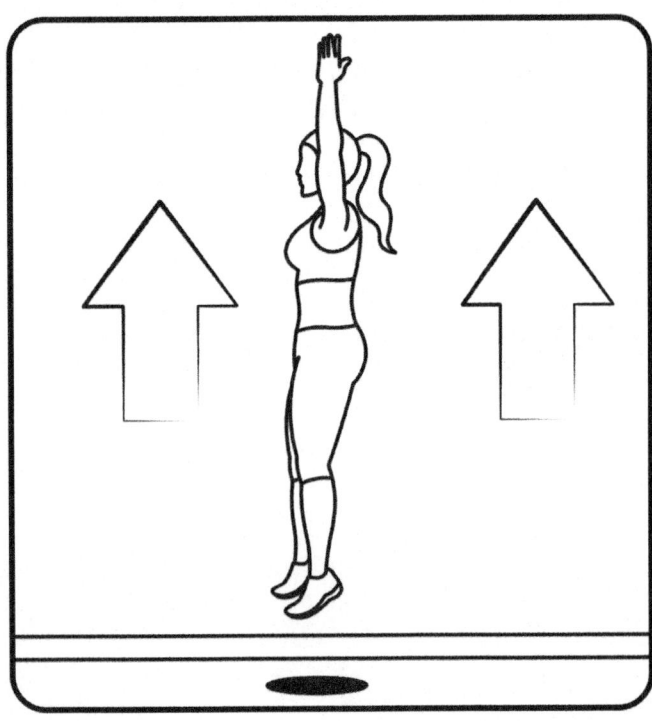

Exercise 5
3-Way Kick

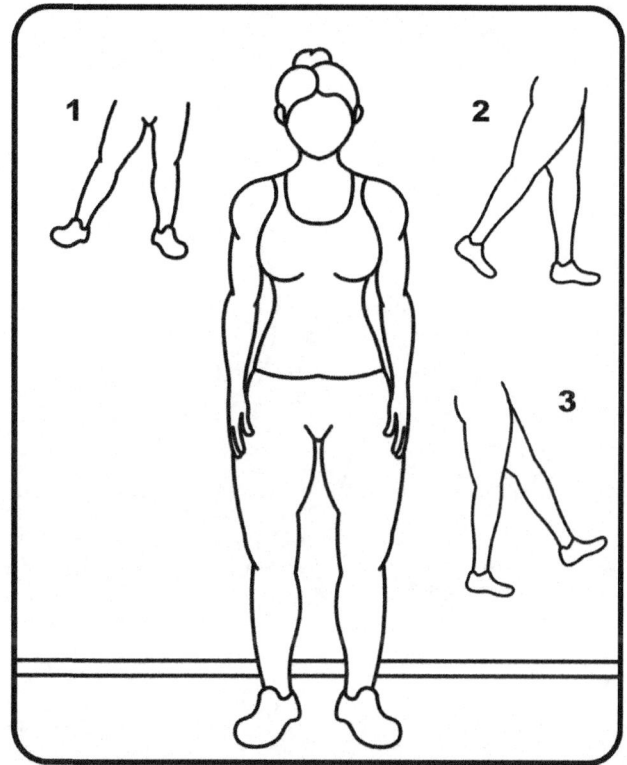

1.) Stand with your feet hip-width apart, and place your hands on your hips.

2.) Shift your weight onto your left foot, and lift your right foot up in front of your body, a few inches from the ground.

3.) Hold your right foot in front of you for 3 seconds, and then bring it down again.

4.) Lift your right foot up to the side of your body, a few inches from the ground, and hold it there for 3 seconds.

5.) Bring your right foot back down under you, and then lift it up behind you, a few inches from the ground, and hold it there for 3 seconds.

6.) Bring your right foot back under you and shift your weight onto your right leg.

7.) Lift your left leg up and repeat these exercises with it. Do this 3 times on each side.

EXERCISE 6
REVERSE LUNGE

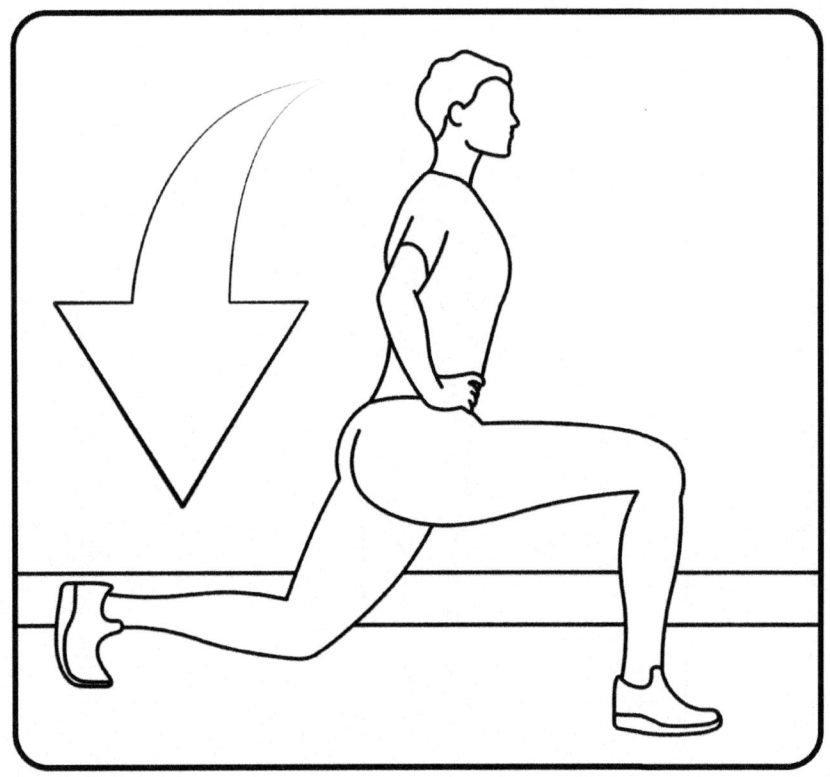

1.) Stand comfortably, with your feet hip-width apart. Place your hands on your hips and spread your weight evenly between your legs.

2.) Move your weight to your left foot, and take your right foot back a large step.

3.) Place the ball of your right foot on the ground and lift your heel up.

4.) Lower your right leg until your thigh is perpendicular with the floor, and your knees are both bent at 90-degree angles.

5.) Press down into your heel and squeeze your glute muscles so that your body lifts back up into your starting position.

6.) Repeat this 5 to 10 times per side.

Exercise 7
Sumo Squats

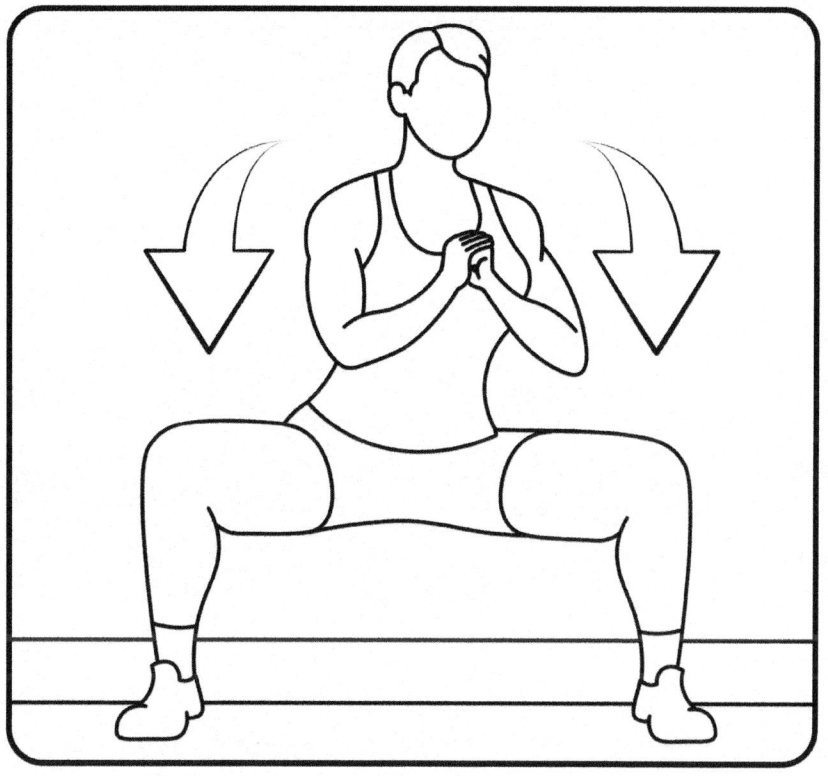

1.) Stand with your feet wide, a little further apart than your shoulders if you can. Your feet should be pointing outwards, at around a 45-degree angle.

2.) Engage your core muscles. Bend your knees and hinge your hips gently to lower into a sumo squat. Move slowly and carefully so you don't hurt yourself.

3.) Spring up quickly, shifting your weight onto your left foot, and lifting until your right foot leaves the ground. Lift your right foot into the air and out to the side.

4.) Lower your right leg back to the floor, and drop back into a squat. Repeat the exercise, but lift your left leg off the floor this time. If you want to increase the difficulty, try holding your leg out to the side for a few seconds, or even pulsing it.

Step by Step Balance-Focused Cardio Exercises for Improved Cardiovascular Health & Stability

Cardio is great for your health, and if you can combine it with balance, you know you're doing well – two benefits for the price of one! You can do some cardio exercises that are great for your balance.

Remember, the point of cardio exercises is to get your heart rate up, so you should aim to do these exercises quickly. You might find that it helps to play some fast-paced music or something similar to help yourself with the pacing. Make sure, though, that you are always in control and you never move so quickly that you feel unsafe.

EXERCISE 1
SIDE STEPPING

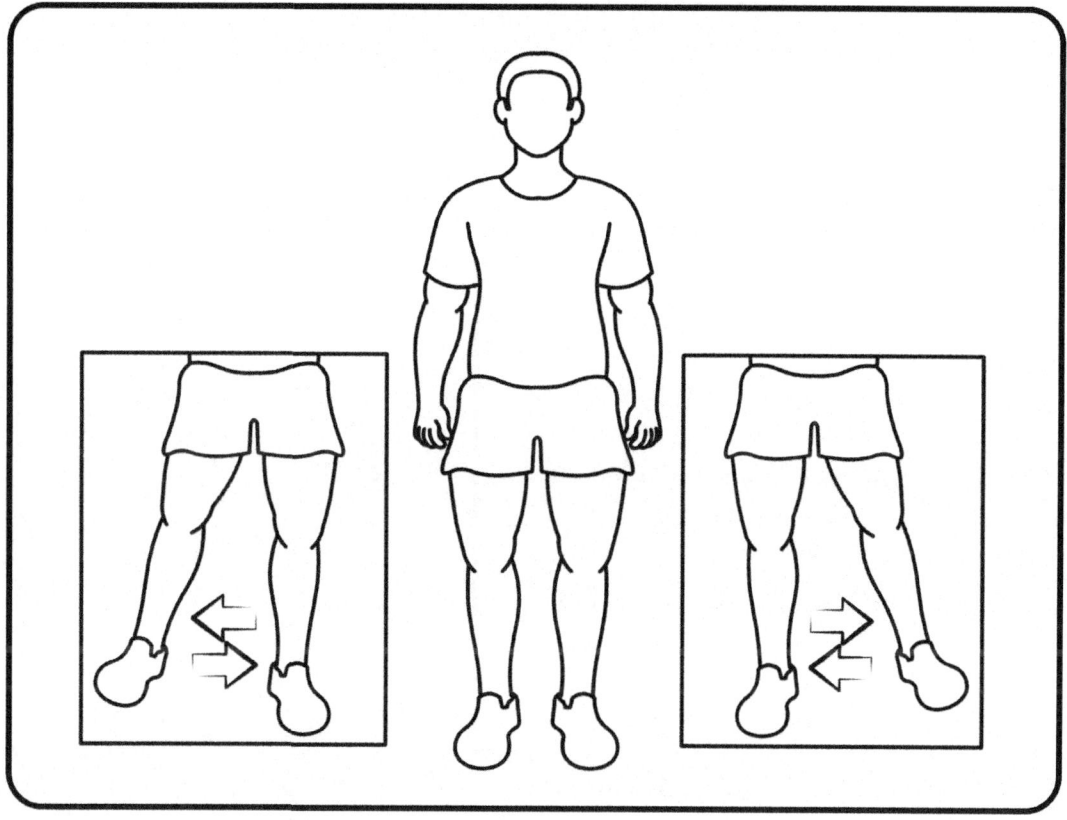

1.) Stand up tall and comfortably, with your chest erect.

2.) Step your right foot out to one side, shifting your weight to your left leg as you do so.

3.) Step your right foot back in, and shift your weight onto your right leg.

4.) Step your left leg out to the side and then bring it back in and shift your weight back onto it.

5.) Move your right foot back out, and continue this pattern for a couple of minutes.

EXERCISE 2
MARCHING ON THE SPOT

1.) Start this exercise by standing up straight on your mat, and then beginning to walk on the spot.

2.) Gradually increase the walking speed, using your arms as well as your legs, so that you are marching on the spot.

3.) Keep your body upright as you walk, making sure you are using all of the muscles in your legs and your abdomen, rather than just your hips.

4.) Keep marching for about 5 minutes, and then relax.

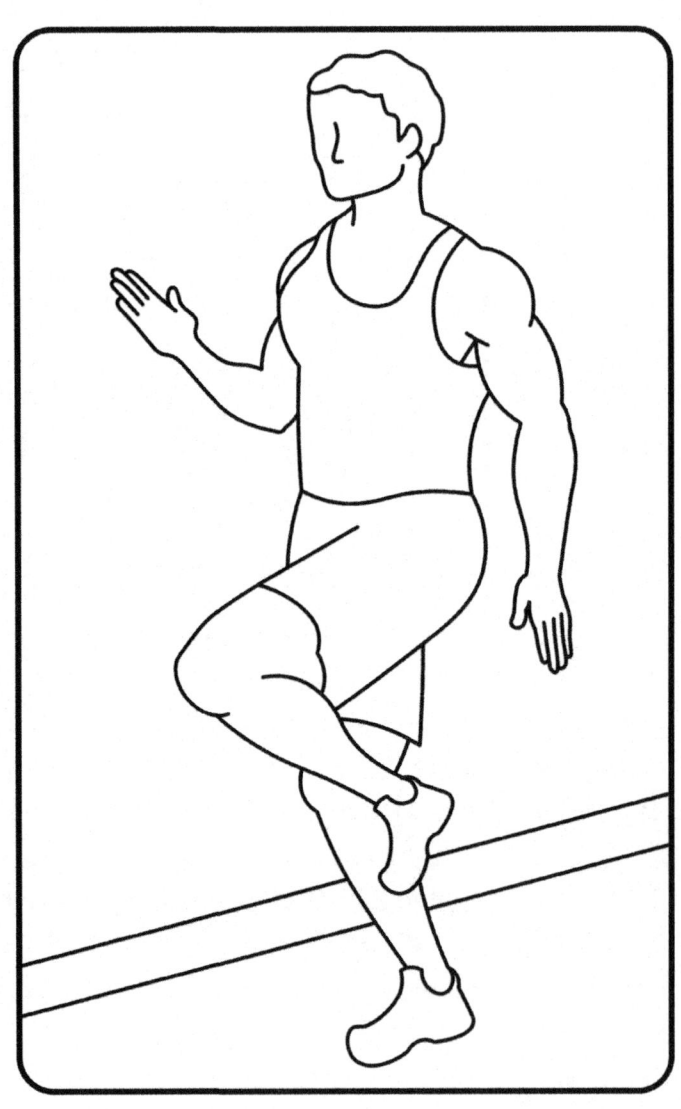

EXERCISE 3
OBLIQUE KNEE LIFTS

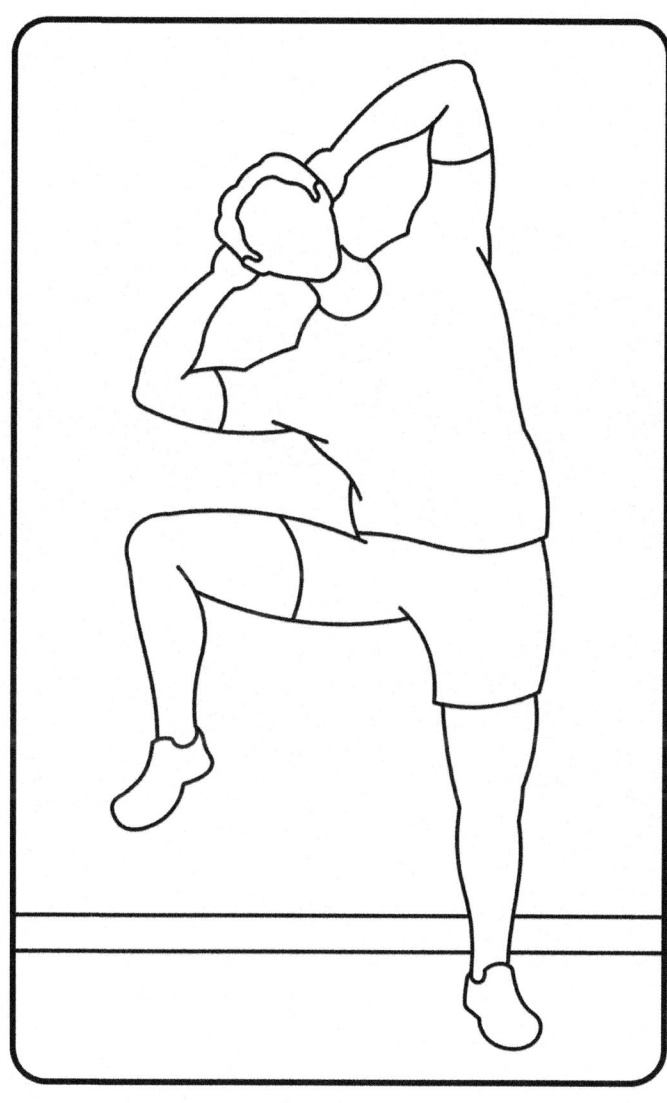

3.) Raise your knee and bring your elbow down towards your knee.

4.) Lift your arm back up and lower your foot towards the floor on your right-hand side.

5.) Bring your knee up and your elbow down.

6.) Repeat this 5 times.

7.) Lower your right foot back to the floor in front of you.

8.) Lift your left arm up over your head, and pick your left foot up, turning your knee out to the side.

9.) Raise your left knee up and lower your left elbow towards your knee.

10.) Lift your left arm back up and lower your foot towards the floor on your left-hand side.

11.) Repeat this 5 times.

1.) Stand up straight, and then lift your right arm up over your head.

2.) Pick your right foot up off the floor, and turn your knee out to the side.

53

EXERCISE 4
RUN AND JUMP

Note: this exercise is quite a difficult one, and does involve jumping. Only perform this if you feel comfortable doing so, and don't push yourself harder than you can cope with. You may hurt yourself otherwise. Make sure you have a flat, comfortable surface and supportive shoes before you attempt it.

1.) Start by marching on the spot, and then pick up the pace so you are running on the spot.

2.) Count to three, and then jump as though you were jumping over something in your path. You can opt for a small jump if you aren't too confident.

3.) As soon as your feet touch the floor, begin running again. Run for a few seconds, and perform another jump.

4.) Keep this up for 3 minutes.

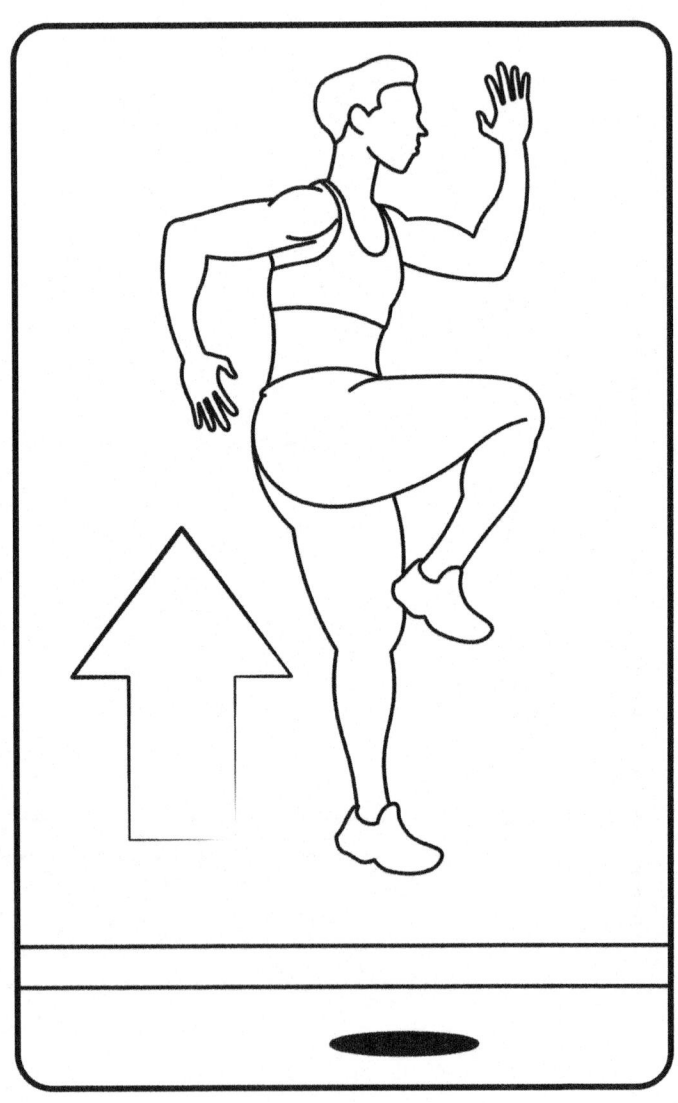

EXERCISE 5
HIP HINGES

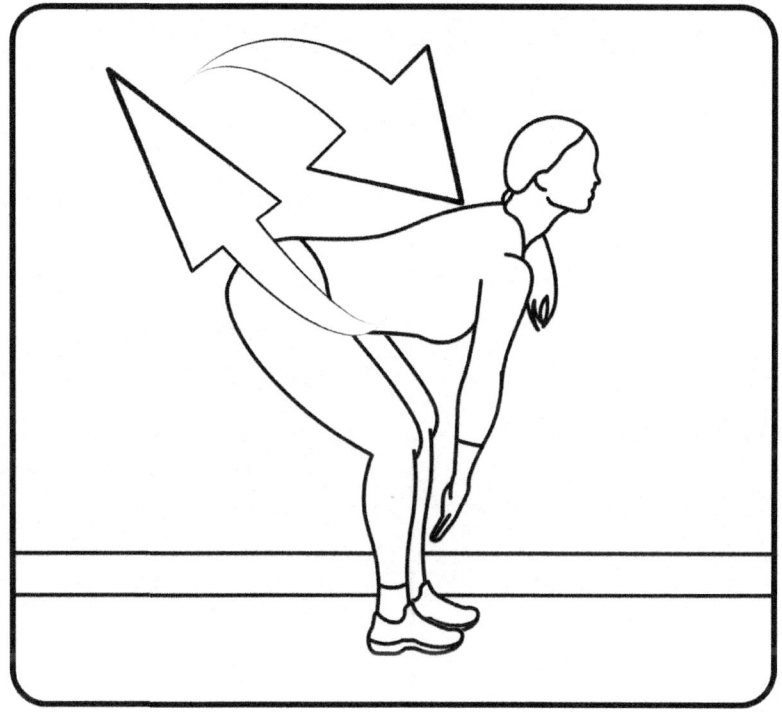

Note: Remember that the goal of cardio is to increase your heart rate. Although you might want to do this exercise slowly to begin with, while you get the feel for it, you should aim to increase so that you are moving quickly, and your blood is pumping. This will ensure you're getting the full benefit of the exercise.

1.) Stand comfortably, with your feet hip-width apart, and your hands resting on your thighs, about halfway down.

2.) Keeping your back flat, hinge at the hips to bend forwards. Slide your hands down your thighs towards your knees as you move. Make sure you don't tip to one side or the other; you want to stay vertical.

3.) Bend until you feel resistance, but keep your back straight, and do not round your spine. You can bend your knees a little if this helps.

4.) Squeeze your glutes and gently push your hips forwards as you come back up to your standing position.

5.) Repeat this 5-10 times.

EXERCISE 6
STEP-UPS

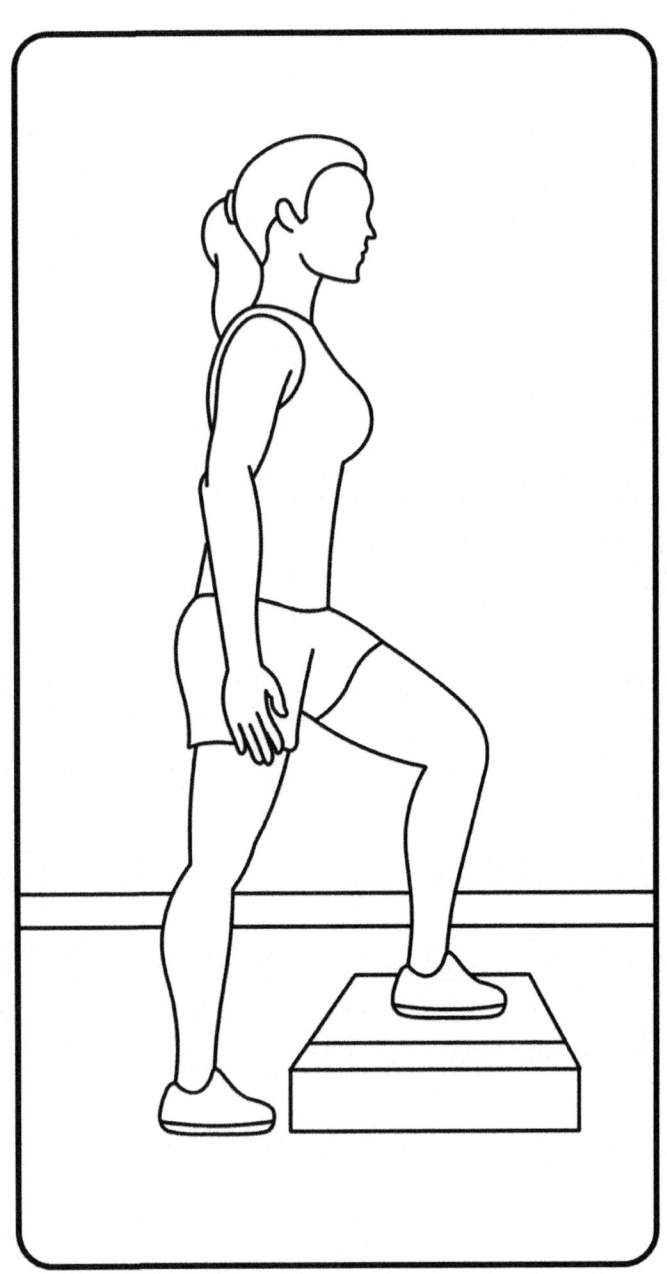

Note: for this exercise, you will need a sturdy step of some sort. A low stool will work as long as it is stable, but you can also use the bottom step of your staircase if that's better. You can grasp the railings if you need support, but try to balance independently if possible.

1.) Stand in front of the step, with your arms at your sides.

2.) Lift your right foot up and onto the step, shifting your weight onto it.

3.) Bring your left leg up to join it.

4.) Step your right leg down again.

5.) Bring your left leg down to join it.

6.) Speed up so you are moving quickly (but not so quickly you become unsafe).

7.) Change directions when you have stepped up 5 times on the right side, and begin stepping up with your left leg first instead. Repeat this 5 times too.

Fall prevention strategies for reducing fall risk in daily life & living safely

As well as the above exercises, you might find it useful to understand some other fall prevention strategies that can help you to stay safe, both when you're at home and when you're out and about.

Fortunately, there are lots of simple things you can do to reduce your risk of falling and hurting yourself. We have already discussed a couple (with the most important one being to see your doctor and find out the cause of balance issues), so let's look at a few others now.

Tip 1) Remove hazards

Although simple, this is a strategy that is very frequently overlooked. Clutter can seriously increase how dangerous your home environment is, especially if it's present in high-traffic areas. Things like dangling cables and cords are particularly hazardous.

You should take some time to clear your home, or get help from a friend or family member if this is difficult for you to do independently. This can involve quite a few different things, but particular areas you should focus on include:

- Securing loose rugs with tape or anti-slip backing (or getting rid of rugs entirely)
- Using non-slip mats where appropriate in the home, especially in the bathroom and near the kitchen sink.
- Clearing high-traffic areas and making sure there is minimal furniture in them.
- Running wires overhead or around the edges of the rooms, rather than across the floors.
- Repairing any damage to your carpets, floors, etc., directly.
- Promptly cleaning up liquids that have been spilled.
- Keeping shoes tidy, so you don't risk tripping when you are entering or leaving your home.

Taking the time to remove hazards from your home can make a significant difference to how confident you feel when moving around. If you have a pet, you may also want to consider strategies to prevent them from getting under your feet, such as training if applicable.

Although you may not be able to remove hazards when you are out and about, you should make a point of noticing them. If you're walking through an area, look out for things that may trip you up, and be careful around them. Pick up your feet when you're walking to avoid tripping on rugs, trailing cables, and steps.

TIP 2) USE LIGHTS

You are at far greater risk of falling if you're operating in a dark environment. A lot of people think that they are familiar enough with their own homes not to worry about this, but many falls occur in the dark. You should take the time to install some extra lights – or brighter lights – around your home.

This is particularly true if you need to get up in the night. Having some dim lights that you leave on at all times to provide a glow if you're moving around in the dark can be crucial. Safety lights that will stay on even in the event of a power cut could also be beneficial.

Make sure there's a lamp within easy reach of your bed or chair, so you can always turn on a light before you stand up. You may also want to add some glow-in-the-dark paint to switches. Always have a light on if you're going to go up or down the stairs.

You should also carry a torch with you when you're out and about (and have one available at home if you frequently get power cuts). You can get pocket torches that will clip onto your keys or fit into a pocket. This can help if you need to navigate somewhere at night.

TIP 3) STAY HYDRATED

Not drinking enough increases your risk of falls, because you may get dizzy if you are dehydrated. It's very easy to underestimate how much you need to drink in a day, so make sure you are drinking enough.

You might want to get a water bottle that tracks how much you drink, or to count the amount your favourite mug holds so you know you're consuming enough liquid. Try to drink throughout the day, not just at the start and the end. Make sure you have a drink with you if you are out and about.

TIP 4) INSTALL RAILS

Although you might not like the idea of having rails in your home, it can be wise to install a few, especially in high-risk places like in the bathroom, or alongside any steps. You might want one near the toilet, or to help yourself in and out of the shower or bath. Having something to hold onto can make you feel more confident. You don't have to use the rails if you don't need them, but having them available may make you feel safer in the home, and could help you to maintain your independence for longer.

You should make sure you use the rails on your staircase (if you have one) too. Stairs are immensely dangerous. According to the Royal Society for the Prevention of Accidents (RoSPA), over 700 people die as a result of falling downstairs each year, and 43,000 people are hospitalised. Always hold on when you are going up or down the steps.

TIP 5) REORGANISE YOUR HOME

It might sound like a lot of hassle to reorganise your home, but doing so can make you safer. You should think about what items you need to use regularly, and make sure that these are as easy as possible to reach.

You are at a much greater risk of falling if you are stretching up to open a cupboard, bending down, or standing on a stool. Although these are good things to practise while exercising, you don't want to have to do them as part of your daily life if you don't feel confident with them.

---

(8) RoSPA. (n.d.). How common are stair-related accidents? Simpson Millar.

https://www.simpsonmillar.co.uk/media/personal-injury/how-common-are-stair-related-accidents/ [accessed 15 May 2023]

You should therefore try to put items that you use frequently within easy reach, and avoid having things you're likely to need in high cupboards. If you do need to reach something from a high cupboard, especially something heavy, get assistance from a neighbour, friend, or family member.

You can reorganise throughout your home, getting clothes that you use regularly within easy reach, and kitchen items within easy reach. Do the same in the bathroom and the rest of your house, and you'll significantly reduce your risk of falls.

TIP 6) PLAN YOUR ROUTES

Preventing falls outside of the home can be harder, because you're more likely to be in an unfamiliar space, and you have less control over your environment. However, it is still possible to increase your safety while you're out and about.

One way you can do this is by planning your routes and knowing where you're going. You can look at Google Street View online to check out the street, and you can call businesses in advance to ask about things like ramps, railings, lifts, etc.

Planning your route also means you'll know how much time to allow for the journey. This can reduce the need to rush somewhere, and you're less likely to fall if you aren't hurrying.

TIP 7) ASK FOR HELP

A lot of people dislike asking for help because they feel like they're being a nuisance, or because they think other people are too busy to help them. However, it's much better to ask for help than to risk hurting yourself, and it's likely that your friends and family would agree.

You can employ this tactic both at home and while out and about. Allow people to help you with things that you find difficult. You may still be able to do the majority of the task yourself, but getting a little assistance can improve your confidence and make you more capable of maintaining your independence.

You might find that you feel safer running errands and attending appointments if somebody goes with you, even if you don't need their assistance. This can help to reduce a fear of falls.

TIP 8) USE AIDS WHEN APPROPRIATE

You might not want to use a cane or a walker, but having one available can be reassuring if you're feeling uncertain. You should accept a walker or a cane if you are offered one, even if you don't plan to use it. You never know when it might help, and it can provide some additional peace of mind to have it available.

These aids can be helpful if you're tired, feeling unsteady after taking medication, under the weather, or otherwise more vulnerable to falls, even if you don't want to use one every day.

TIP 9) AVOID SLIPPERY SOCKS

Some people dislike wearing shoes and prefer to move around their homes in socks only. This can be more comfortable and might seem harmless, but it can significantly increase your risk of falls, especially when you're on hard floors. Kitchen and bathroom floors are often tiled, which makes them slippery, and this presents a significant fall risk.

It's much better to either go barefoot, or to wear shoes if you're walking on slippery surfaces. Socks reduce your friction and allow you to slide around too much. You're likely to go flying at some stage, whether that's as you turn around to do something, or hurry to answer the phone.

We mentioned getting comfortable but well-fitted shoes above – but wearing them in the home (as well as when you go out) is key to protecting yourself from falls.

It's also worth noting that you should think about your clothing choices in general. Avoid wearing clothes that trail beneath your feet or that fit badly, and make sure any shoelaces are tied, so there's no risk of you standing on them.

Tip 10) Consider home adaptations

Home adaptations doesn't have to be as drastic as it might sound, and some local councils will cover certain adaptations so you don't have to pay for the costs.

The adaptations that are available and useful to you can vary from person to person, but might include things like fitting grab rails or lowering your kitchen counters to make things easier to reach. Get in touch with your local council to find out more about the things that will help to reduce your risk of falls at home.

Tip 9) Avoid slippery socks

Some people dislike wearing shoes and prefer to move around their homes in socks only. This can be more comfortable and might seem harmless, but it can significantly increase your risk of falls, especially when you're on hard floors. Kitchen and bathroom floors are often tiled, which makes them slippery, and this presents a significant fall risk.

It's much better to either go barefoot, or to wear shoes if you're walking on slippery surfaces. Socks reduce your friction and allow you to slide around too much. You're likely to go flying at some stage, whether that's as you turn around to do something, or hurry to answer the phone.

We mentioned getting comfortable but well-fitted shoes above – but wearing them in the home (as well as when you go out) is key to protecting yourself from falls.

It's also worth noting that you should think about your clothing choices in general. Avoid wearing clothes that trail beneath your feet or that fit badly, and make sure any shoelaces are tied, so there's no risk of you standing on them.

Step by Step Advanced Exercises to Improve Stability and Balance

Before we finish up, you might want some more challenging exercises to try. Bear in mind that these exercises are designed for those who have quite good levels of physical ability, and they may be riskier than the others we have covered so far. If you are going to attempt them, make sure you prioritise safety, and don't push beyond your comfort levels. You need to be careful and make sure you're not putting yourself in danger.

All of the below exercises will help you to improve your balance and stability, but you may want to try them when you have already practised some of the others contained in this book.

Make sure you are wearing comfortable, supportive shoes, and working in a safe space. Always have a backup plan for if you fall over and need to call for assistance – don't exercise without one.

Exercise 1
Stretched Limbs

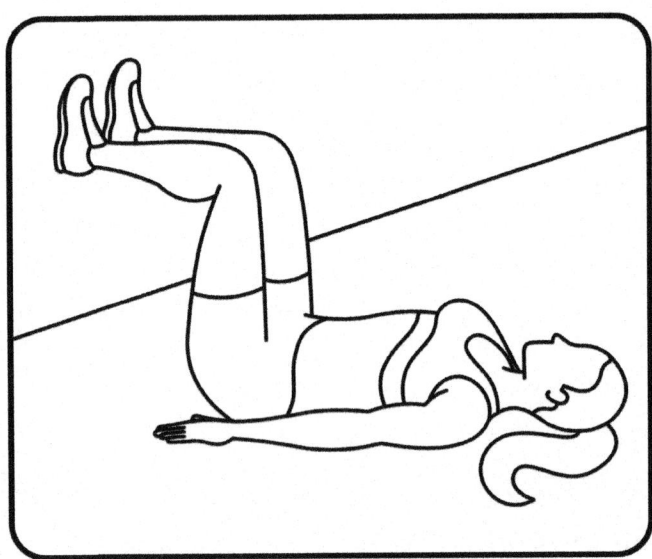 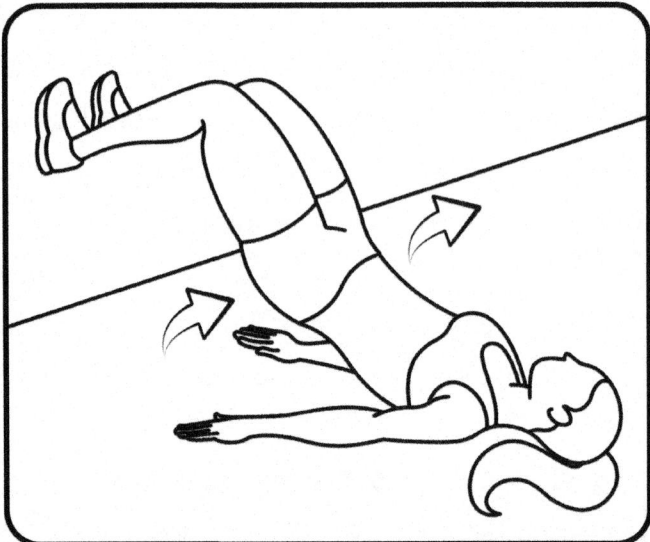

1.) Start on a flat surface with a clear area both ahead and behind you. Take a deep breath, and stretch your arms up above your head.

2.) Hinge at the hips, keeping your arms above your head and your back straight, so that the top of your body becomes horizontal, and you're looking at the floor with your arms stretched forwards.

3.) Once you are stable, lift your right leg off the floor and extend it out behind you, lifting it as high as you can. The goal is to get your right leg, back, and arms all in a line with each other, parallel to the floor. Your weight will all be on your left leg. It may take some practise to achieve this.

4.) Hold the position for 20 seconds if you can, and then lower your leg back to the floor in a controlled fashion, and straighten up from your hips.

5.) Swap sides, and repeat the exercise with your left leg off the floor.

6.) Repeat this on both sides 5 times, and then return to a standing position.

Exercise 2
Single Leg Squat

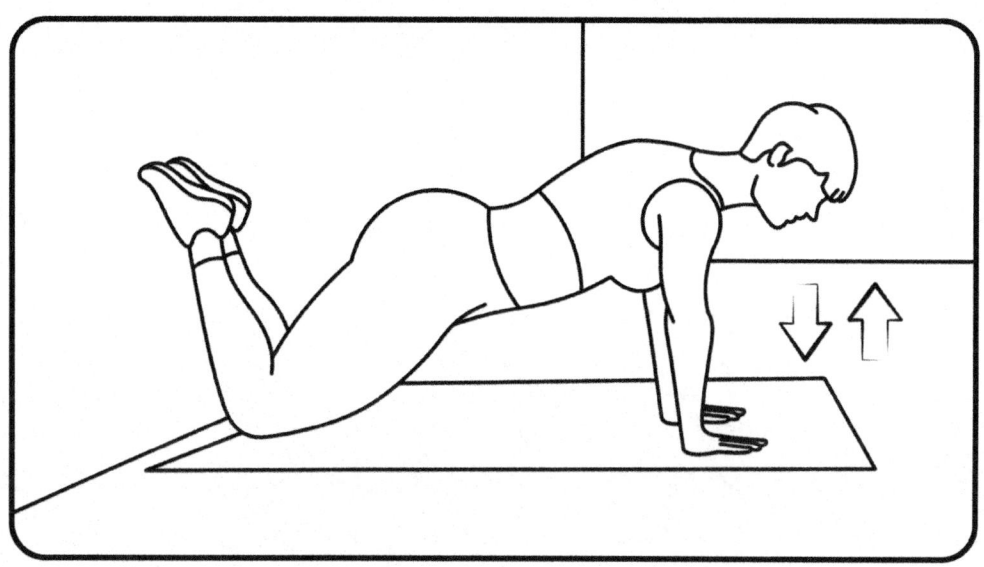

1.) Stand up straight on a flat surface. Have a wall or chair nearby that you can put your hand on if you need to.

2.) Shift your weight onto your left leg, and gradually lift your right foot off the ground, keeping your right leg straight.

3.) Start to bend your left leg, squatting down a few inches. Make sure your knee is in line with your toes, and doesn't bend to one side or the other.

4.) Squat down a few inches, and then straighten back up into the upright position.

5.) Repeat this 5 times on your left leg, and then swap sides and do 5 squats with your right leg. Remember to keep your knee over your toes, so you don't pull any muscles.

EXERCISE 3
TIGHTROPE WALK

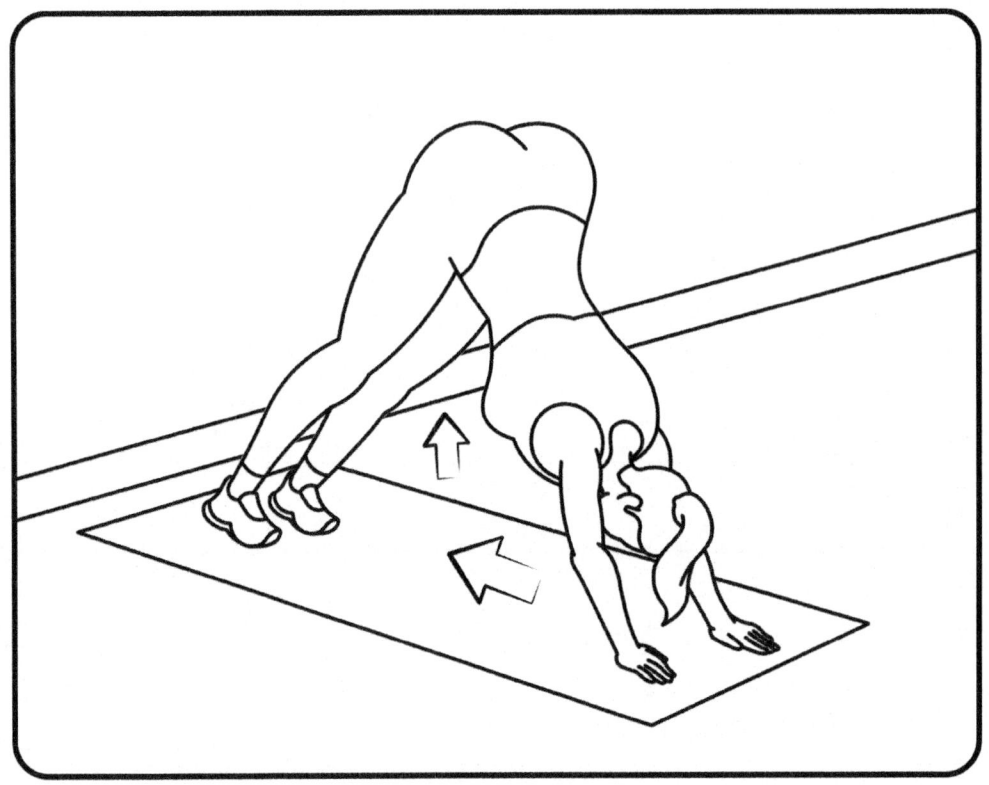

Note: For this exercise, you will need to lie a piece of string straight along the floor. The longer the piece of string, the more challenging the exercise will be.

1.) Set your piece of string on the floor in a straight line across the room.

2.) Start from one end. Place your right foot on the piece of string, and then begin to walk along it, placing your feet directly in front of each other, on top of the string.

3.) Walk at least 15 paces like this if you are able to.

4.) Turn around and walk in the other direction, this time leading with your left foot.

EXERCISE 4
TREE MOVEMENTS

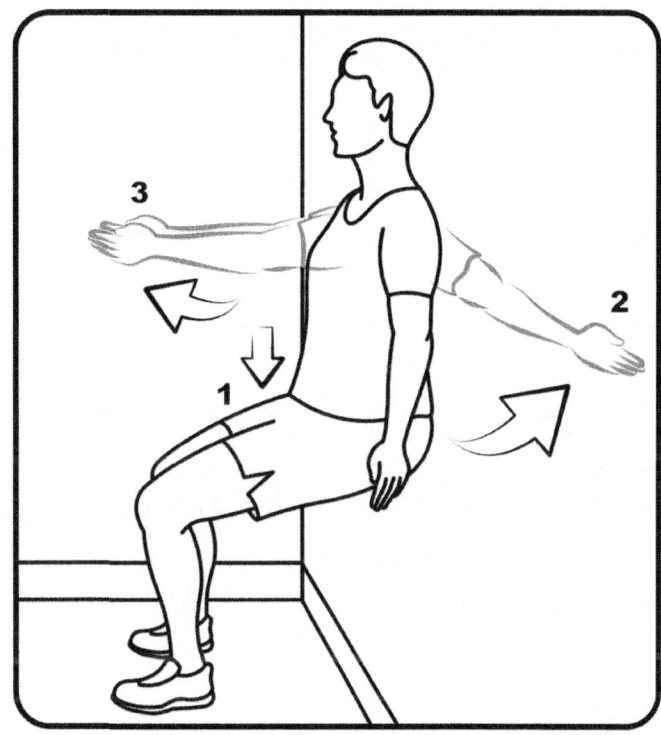

1.) Stand with your toes touching each other, and your heels a short distance apart.

2.) Lift your toes off the floor and spread them out, engaging the muscles in your lower legs.

3.) Activate the muscles in your core and hold them taut as you slightly bend your knees.

4.) Gradually shift your weight to your left foot, and press the inner edge of your foot against the floor.

5.) Lift your right leg up and bend the right knee, so your ankle is elevated. Place the sole of your right foot against your left thigh (or your left calf if this is too challenging). Don't place it against your left knee, as this can destabilise you.

6.) Turn your toes towards the floor, and count to 30 in this position if you are able to.

7.) Return your right foot to the floor, and then repeat this exercise on your left-hand side by lifting your left leg up and placing your foot against your right thigh (or calf).

Exercise 5
Clock Turns

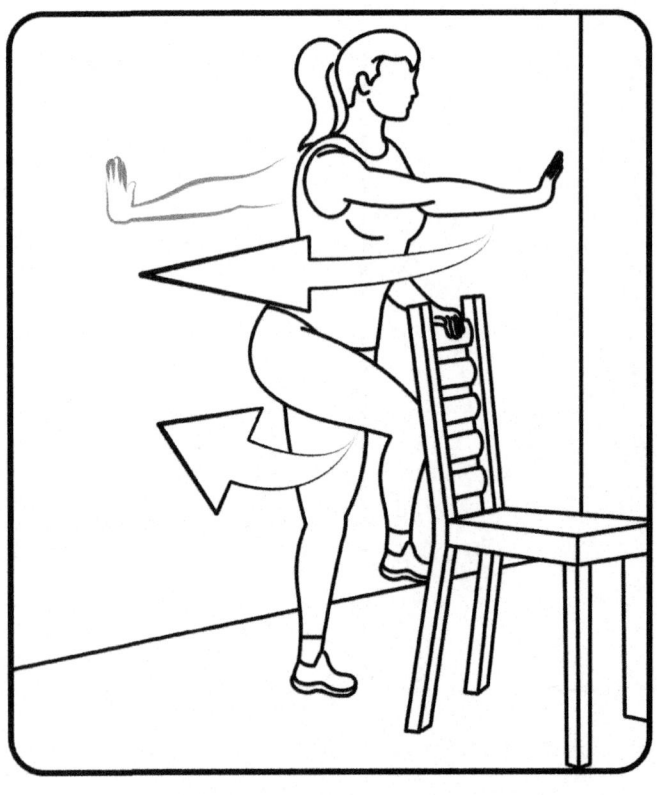

4.) Keeping your foot up and your face pointing forwards, slowly turn your arm to the side, as though it was pointing to the number 3.

5.) Still looking forwards and keeping your foot in the air, gradually turn your arm behind you, to point at the number 6.

6.) Slowly bring your arm back to the number 3, and then back to the number 12, still looking in front of you.

7.) Put your foot on the floor and swap so that you have lifted up your left leg and your left arm.

8.) Repeat this exercise 3 times on each side.

Note: You may find that it helps to use a chair for support when you first attempt this exercise. You can place the hand you aren't using on the back of the chair. Aim to become independent of the chair eventually.

1.) Stand up straight and comfortably, with your feet hip-width apart.

2.) Imagine that you are facing the number 12 on a clock. The number 6 is directly behind you.

3.) Lift up your right leg and stretch your right arm out in front of you, as though you were pointing at the number 12.

Exercise 6
Wall Push-Ups

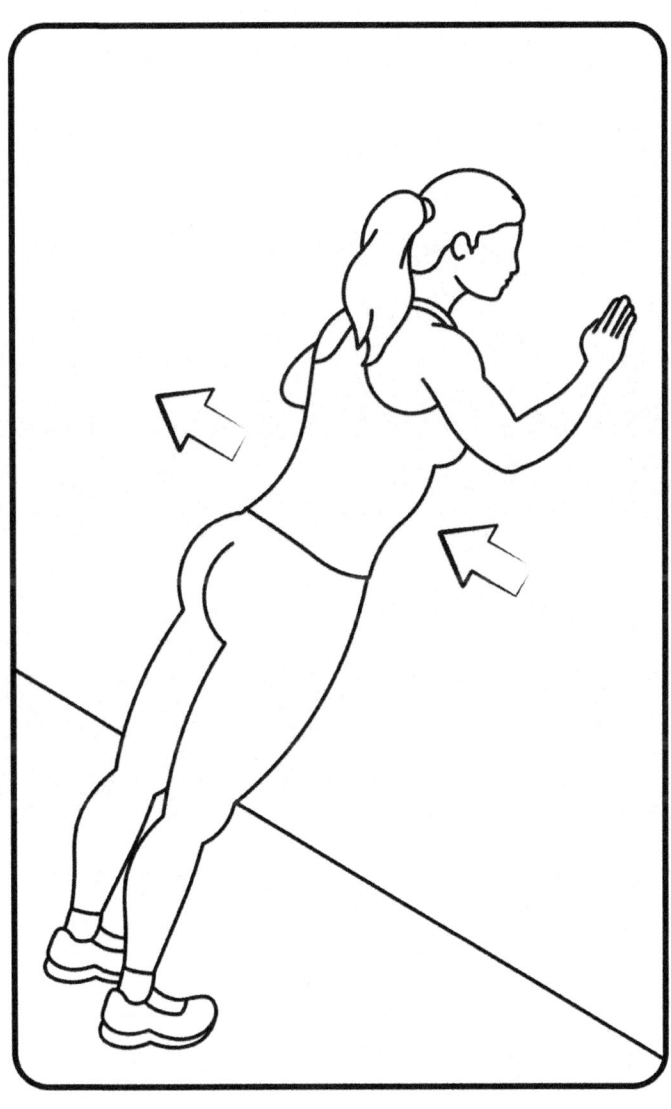

1.) Face the wall. Start in a standing position, with your feet hip-width apart.

2.) Lift your arms so that your hands are positioned slightly below your shoulders, the palms facing outwards, towards the wall.

3.) Step your feet back a little way so your body is at a slight angle, and put your weight on your hands, so your body forms a straight line between your feet and the top of your head.

4.) Brace your abs and glutes, and begin lowering your elbows towards the wall, so your body approaches the wall.

5.) When you have reached the wall, press with your hands to push your body away, keeping your back straight as you move.

6.) Lower back towards the wall, making sure you stay in control of the movement. Repeat this 5 times.

Note: you will find this exercise easier to complete if you have a blank wall you can use.

EXERCISE 7
BACK LEG LIFT

Note: You again may want a chair for this exercise initially, but you should aim to perform it without eventually.

1.) Stand facing the back of the chair. Shift your weight onto your left leg.

2.) Gradually lift your right leg up behind you, keeping your knee straight and your foot angled as though you were still standing on it. Don't point your toes.

3.) Lift your right leg as far as you can without bending it, and then hold this position for up to 10 seconds.

4.) Gently lower your foot back to the floor. Repeat this exercise 3 times on this side, and then swap legs.

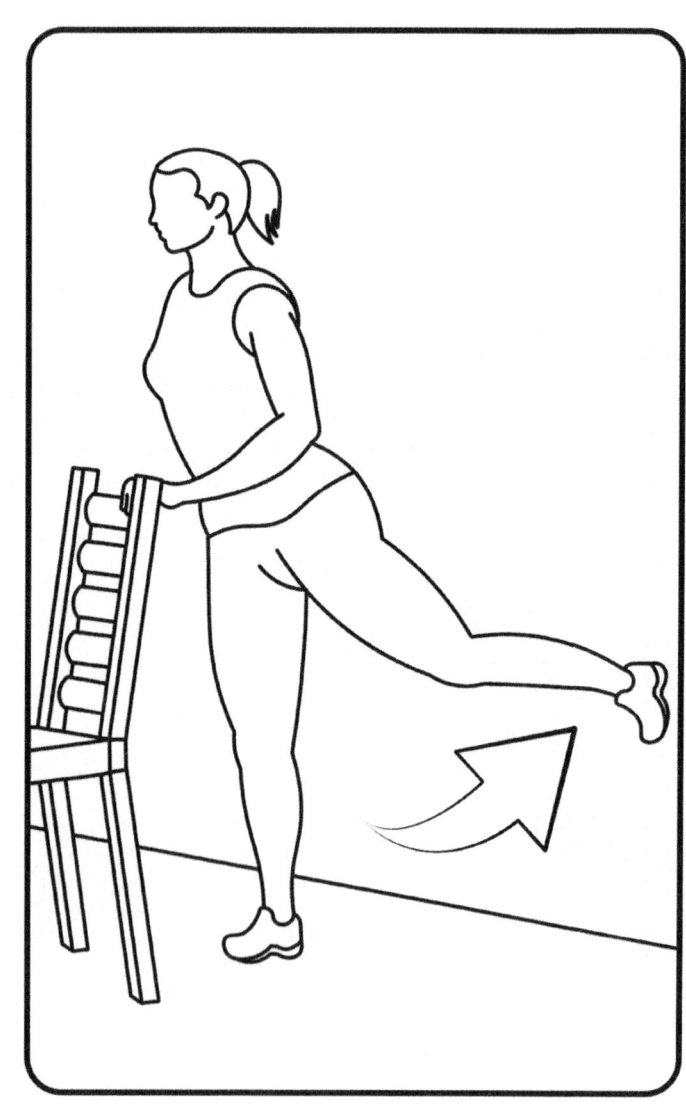

70

Progression and maintenance strategies to keep going & stick to your new habits

Hopefully, you've now got some great techniques for improving your balance and stability, and for increasing your confidence in yourself. However, there is one thing left to do: make sure you stick to these strategies!

It can be difficult to maintain an exercise routine once you've started one, and often, people slip backwards just when they think they've mastered it. Forming new habits is hard, and you might find that although you exercise thoroughly for a few days or weeks, you soon stop practising, and your balance starts to deteriorate again.

It's very easy to do this, unfortunately, and it happens to a lot of people. You might feel enthusiastic to begin with, but then you slide backwards and stop practising entirely.

That's why we're going to finish off by looking at a few top tips to help ensure you stay on track with your new exercise routine and continue to improve your balance.

Tip 1) Set a dedicated time

Even if you've retired, finding the time to exercise can be a big challenge. The days often seem too full, but you need to make space if you want to see improvements in your balance. Most people find that it helps to have a dedicated time of day in which they exercise. It's a good idea to do this when you're feeling fresh and energetic, and not worn out. You're much less likely to be able to balance well – or to feel like trying – if you're already tired.

You may therefore want to put this exercise slot somewhere in the morning or afternoon, depending on your energy levels and other commitments. You might, for example, decide you will do 10 minutes of balancing after breakfast. It may be a good idea to give your brain some time to wake up first, as some people feel light-headed and disorientated when they first wake up, and need a bit of time to come round.

Whenever you decide to do it, try to clear your schedule at that time so you can be consistent. Sometimes, this may not be possible, but the more you do it, the more benefits you will gain. If you already exercise at a regular time, you may want to simply incorporate balancing into your routine, but if not, you can start a routine with balance.

TIP 2) HAVE A DEDICATED AREA

The chances of you reliably exercising if you have a cluttered and unusable area are much slimmer. You should make a dedicated space, and keep it clear and tidy. This makes exercise far more accessible, and vastly increases the chances of you doing it.

For example, if you decide you are going to exercise in your living room, you should make sure that the space is clear before your exercise slot rolls around. If you have to clear the space as well as exercise, you're much more likely to decide that it's too much work, and to delay it – or to get distracted by cleaning and fail to practise.

When you're working on improving your balance, having a clear and comfortable space is crucial. You need to be able to put your hand on a wall or a sturdy chair when necessary, and you need to be able to lift and move your legs and arms around freely, without bumping into things. You can't practise safely if the space isn't open.

If the area is clear and free when the time to practise rolls around, you're far more likely to actually exercise than if it's cluttered.

TIP 3) SET SOME GOALS

It's hard to keep exercising if you don't get any sense of progress or of why you're doing it. You are much more likely to find you can maintain your daily exercise if you are reminded about why you are doing it, and you feel like you're getting somewhere. Aim to have some small goals you are always working towards. For example, a goal could be to feel comfortable walking across your garden without your stick, or to know you can get up from your chair without assistance or difficulty.

Keep a written note of these goals so you can have the pleasure of ticking them off as you achieve them. This should make it easier to feel a sense of progress, because you can easily review your whole journey.

It's a good idea to have both short-term goals and some long-term goals, so you've got some things to work on immediately, and a sense of where you're going in the future.

TIP 4) REWARD YOURSELF

Everybody likes a reward when they have done something well, and this is a good way to make a habit stick. Try to find some small reward that you can give yourself, either after an exercise session, or when you have achieved one of your goals.

Rewards don't need to be big or expensive, but they should be something that you can look forward to. For example, you might allow yourself to watch your favourite TV show, read a few pages of your favourite book, or have a sweet treat with a cup of tea or coffee when you've done your exercises. This is a great way to make sure you associate exercise with something positive, which makes you much more likely to do it.

TIP 5) DON'T GO FOR ALL-OR-NOTHING

Some people take a very hardline approach to exercise and think that if they aren't going to do their full workout, it's not worth doing anything. This sort of thinking, more often than not, leads to doing nothing – which obviously isn't a good idea.

You should instead take a "some is better than none" approach. If you haven't got time to do a half-hour workout, fit in ten minutes, and be proud of those ten minutes. You don't have to always meet your exact goals to be making progress. You haven't failed if you have to adjust your exercise routine and take a different approach to it.

Tip 6) Get help

Some people find that they exercise a lot better when they have external input. You may not be hitting the gym with your closest friends anymore, but that doesn't mean nobody can help you with your balance exercises. There are various ways that you can use the input of others to make sure you keep exercising. One option is to take a weekly class; this injects structure and discipline into your routine, and also offers some valuable social aspects too.

However, that won't be an option for everyone, so think outside the box. Could you meet a friend in a park to do some balance exercises together? Have somebody drop by in the evenings to do them with you?

Another option is to have a family member call to check whether you've done your exercises. This is a different kind of support, but it may provide you with the push you need to keep exercising every day. You could also consider exercising to YouTube videos or workout DVDs. Although this is not the same as having somebody with you in person, it can still help to make exercise feel more sociable and enjoyable.

Tip 7) Take breaks

It might sound counter-intuitive to take time off when you're trying to get a habit to stick, and it's true that you should use this tip with caution, but taking a break when you need one is key. When you're feeling burnt out, either physically or mentally, a break is crucial to resetting and getting yourself back on track.

It's fine to take a day or two when you simply decide that you aren't going to exercise. As long as you get back on track after the break, this can be beneficial for your mind and your body, and it can make it easier to cement your balance exercises as a regular part of your routine. Rest days are important. Hopefully, you now have some great tips to help you stay on track and achieve your exercise goals! Remember, if you do get into a rut and stop for a while, you can always start again later.

Printed in Great Britain
by Amazon

38081910R00044